MENIERE'S I
THE REAL STORY

THIS BOOK IS DEDICATED
TO ALL WHO ARE AFFLICTED
WITH MENIERE'S DISEASE,
THEIR FAMILIES, FRIENDS,
AND ALL WHO SUFFER WITH
THEM.

Ménière's Disease. The Real Story.
Printed by: Optichrome Ltd., 98 Maybury Road,
Woking, Surrey, GU21 5HX.
Published by, and Copyright held by:
Ménière's Society, 98 Maybury Road,
Woking, Surrey, GU21 5HX.
First Published: March 1992
ISBN 0 9519301 0 9

MENIERE'S DISEASE

THE REAL STORY

DISCLAIMER

Whilst every effort has been made to secure accuracy, the Ménière's Society expressly disclaims liability to any person for carrying out any of the regimes referred to in this book. Much of the content is personal experiences of sufferers and should only be regarded as such.

NO PERSON SHOULD CHANGE THEIR MEDICAL TREATMENT WITHOUT FIRST CONSULTING THEIR DOCTOR.

compiled and edited by
JOHN MYALL and TERRY SHEPPARD

ACKNOWLEDGEMENTS:

Our special thanks to:-
Optichrome Ltd.,
98 Maybury Road,
Woking, Surrey,
GU21 5HX.

who have continually provided so much support and assistance for the Ménière's Society and, help towards the production of this book, and to:-

Duphar Laboratories Ltd.,
Gaters Hill, West End,
Southampton, Hants.,
SO3 3JD.

for their continued interest in the Ménière's Society for sponsoring this book, their encouragement and un-stinting assistance.

.....and to all of the sufferers and members of the medical profession for their contributions. We are well aware that it has been difficult for some sufferers, physically and mentally, to relay their experiences to us. Equally, we are grateful to the doctors for taking time out to provide us with material specifically for "The Book". We do appreciate how precious time is to them.

CONTENTS

NOTES FROM THE EDITORS

A big "thank you" to all who have sent in contributions and ideas for this book. Without you it would not have been possible.

There were many contributions that were worthy of publication but were omitted simply through lack of space. Do not be disheartened, if this book is the success we think it will be, there may be a volume two....

Only if the writer specifically stated that we may print their name in full have we done so. In all other cases the articles are identified only by the author's initials and an abbreviated address.

. . .

The effects of Ménière's disease can be unpredictable and diverse, the sufferers themselves coping in different ways. Equally, it is well understood that many so called 'diagnosed' cases are not genuine sufferers. It is very difficult to assess the success of conventional or alternative regimes because of the episodic nature of the condition, giving rise to false results in any trials.

INTRODUCTION

The origins of this book date back to 1984 when a friend informed me that one day I would write a book about Ménière's disease. The author of very good books herself such as "Deafness in the Adult", Winifred Brinson was quite sure, even then, of the eventuality of this book. I have to say that as camping is my one passion and since I have had several abortive attempts at writing a book on the subject, I was not so sure about taking on a second book.

As members of the Society sent in their stories to me, I began to realise the possibility of producing a book but written by the sufferers themselves. There are many books on the subject of Ménière's disease but none that I could find designed towards the actual sufferer as the reader. Relevant books tend to be too complicated for the general public to understand, the content therein being aimed towards members of the medical profession. Hopefully, all can enjoy and learn from this book.

Lastly, I must thank John Myall. Not only a long term volunteer in the office but a good friend and mentor. Severe hearing loss renders the telephone a difficult "accessory" thus ending his potential as a Samaritan but with the help of hearing aids and lip-reading, he is still a good "listener". I have off-loaded many of my problems onto him including much of the work required to ensure the production of this book.

Terry Sheppard
Co-Ordinator. Ménière's Society

CHAPTER ONE

PROSPER MENIERE

PROSPER MENIERE (1799 - 1862)

by

Andrew Morrison FRCS

Chairman - Medical Advisory Committee

Prosper Ménière was born in the Loire Valley at Angers on 18th June 1799, the son of a merchant, Louis-Prosper Ménière. In the same year Napoleon Bonaparte had become First Consul of France, later Emperor. When Ménière was 14 years old, Britain and her allies took Paris and banished Napoleon to Elba. The final French defeat at Waterloo, a year later, resulted in Napoleon's abdication and imprisonment on St. Helena island, with restoration of the monarchy under Louis XVIII.

After studying the classics and botany he became a medical student at the Hotel Dieu in Angers and in 1819 moved to the sister hospital in Paris. He was awarded the Gold Medal in 1826 and his Doctorate in 1828.

Following the death of Louis XVIII in 1824, his surviving brother became Charles X. Charles was an unpopular king who, following the insurrection of 1830, was forced to abdicate. In the summer of 1830, Ménière was a clinical assistant to Dupuytren. He recorded the reactions of the excitable Parisians and gave graphic accounts of the animated scenes at the Hotel Dieu where hundreds of casualties were treated. Ménière's life and career were soon destined to become involved in, and influenced by, the Bourbon descendants of Charles X.

In 1830, Louis Phillippe became King of France. For nearly 18 years France prospered under this "Citizen King". During this time of relative tranquillity Ménière's academic career advanced from strength to strength. When cholera broke out, he worked in an improvised department in the Arsenal and wrote daily of his terrible experiences. In the same year, 1832, he was made Professor Agrégé of the Faculty, nominated surgeon of the Fourth Dispensary of the Philanthropic Society and of the Relief Committee of the XIth District of Paris.

The second son of Charles X, the Duc de Berri, had been assassinated in 1820. His widow, the Duchess Caroline Louise, had borne a son, the Duc de Bordeaux. In 1832, the Duchess conspired to regain the throne for her son. The attempt failed and she was imprisoned at Blaye. In 1833, Ménière was appointed to the Citadel of Blaye in the service of the Duchess de Berri. He supervised her pregnancy and the birth of her daughter, gained her confidence and ascertained that she had secretly married the Italian Count Lucchesi-Palli. The release of this information lost the Duchess all support in France and ingratiated Ménière with the establishment. Ménière spent about a year in the service of the Duchess, who revived his great interest in Botany.

On returning to Paris in 1834, Ménière worked in Dr. Chomel's department and in 1835 was sent into the Department d'Aude and the Haute Garonne to organise health care against cholera. For this work he gained the chevalier of the Legion d'Honneur and in 1837 was appointed Professor of the Faculty of Hygiene. His thesis for the Chair of Hygiene was on "clothes and cosmetics".

The following year he married the daughter of Becquerel, a member of the Institute of Deaf Mutes in Paris and in the same year was appointed Doctor in Chief of this Institute. His son, Emile, was born the following year. Thereafter, Ménière largely neglected his academic teaching and his interest in military practice in favour of his passion for botany and his increasing involvement in diseases of the ear. He lived with his father-in-law and spent much of his time in the Botanical Gardens. He moved in Parisian society and was a friend of Honore de Balzac, Franz Liszt and Victor Hugo.

During the 1840s Louis Phillippe became less of a Citizen's King, developing reactionary tendencies, tampering with justice and interfering with the freedom of the Press. In 1848 there was a general left-wing revolutionary movement which affected almost every European state. The Marx and Engels Communist Manifesto was published that year. The Revolution of 1848 succeeded in France, Louis Phillippe fled to England, the French Republic was proclaimed and Bonaparte's nephew became President of France, later the Emperor Napoleon III.

In the Spring of 1848 Ménière wrote counter revolutionary articles every two weeks, anonymously, in a Parisienne Review. Despite legal action against the journal, the identity of the mysterious correspondent of "Republic in 1848" remained secret until many years later. This seems to have been Ménière's last attempt to influence the political scene.

In 1848 Ménière published a French translation from the German textbook by Kramer, "Treatise on Diseases of the Ear" with his own notes and numerous additions. One of these additions is considered to have been the first description of Ménière's disease. Translated into English it read as follows:-

> "I have seen a young girl afflicted with sudden deafness, total deafness which occurred in the short space of a few hours. Travelling in an open carriage and exposed during particularly cold night while menstruating, she lost her

> hearing although no pain was felt in either ear. Her death which promptly followed, allowed me to dissect with care the two temporal bones, and I found in the whole labyrinth a sort of plastic, reddish lymph which appeared to cover all the surface membrane and covering the internal ear."

This fatal illness, whatever the cause, was not due to the condition which we know as idiopathic Ménière's disease.

Ménière remained Chief of the Institute of Deaf Mutes from his appointment in 1838 until his death 27 years later. During this time his interests were diverse. His publications and writings are too numerous to itemize; they include literary fantasies, and works on medicine, philosophy, horticulture and botany. In 1856 he became a Vice President of the Botanical Society.

On 8th January 1861, when Prosper Ménière presented his short paper to the Paris Academy of Medicine, it was violently opposed. In an era when patients with this disease were considered to be suffering from variants of epilepsy or of apoplexy, Ménière's great contribution was to draw attention to the inner ear as a source of the diverse symptoms and signs of the condition which bears his name.

Following Ménière's first paper, Trousseau, then Chief of the Hotel Dieu, presented his opposing views on the epileptic nature of the disease, and Ménière countered with further papers supporting his conditions. Heated controversy on many aspects of this bewildering disease continue to this day.

In an era when more scientific assessment was not possible, Ménière listened to his patients and came to his conclusions from astute observation. The following excerpt from one of his papers emphasises this point:-

> "There came to my attention some time ago, a number of patients with a series of symptoms which were always the same. Symptoms which appeared serious and gave the impression of an organic lesion of the worst kind, recurring from time to time, from week to week, from month to month or from year to year.
>
> A young healthy man experiences, for no apparent reason, vertigo, nausea and vomiting, an inexpressibly distressing state takes all his strength away, his pale face bathed with sweat suggests he is about to faint. Often the patient, after feeling unsteady, falls dazed to the ground without being able to get up and lying on his back is unable to open his eyes without seeing surrounding objects spinning around him. The slightest movement of his head makes the vertigo and nausea worse and the vomiting starts again as soon as the patient tries to change position. Incidents of the same kind recurred frequently causing serious anxiety especially as between each crisis he was inclined to vertigo and deafness. The patient could not move his head suddenly, turn to right or to left without losing his balance; his gait became unsteady, he veered involuntarily to one side and the ground appeared uneven - sudden movements resulted in functional disorders of this kind. If the patient when he was lying down moved suddenly into a horizontal position, immediately the bed and all the surrounding objects began spinning, he felt as if he

was on a ship on the high seas and became nauseated. If he got up suddenly into a vertical position exactly the same phenomena occurred, and if he tried to walk, he would immediately fall down.

Other doctors saw this as cerebral congestion necessitating a rigorous regime of blood-letting and purging, but experience proved that this treatment, though followed with extreme rigour, remained ineffective and the prognosis remained very bad.

The patient continued to complain of other symptoms. For example, noises in his ears, often very loud and very persistent, and a noticeable hearing loss on one side and sometimes even on both sides and it was because of this that a doctor specializing in ear disease was called in. I examined the organs and did not discover the slightest trace of a lesion but I noted the relation between the deafness and the 'cerebral troubles'. I have frequently seen similar cases and I became interested in researching them further. I came to the conclusion that these cerebral and auditory lesions were a single illness.

With patients who were good historians, it was possible for me, by dint of very careful questioning, to establish that the vertigo, the faintness, the sudden falling down and the vomiting, had been preceded by noises in the ears which occurred for no apparent reason and, which persisted during attacks and, that they coincided often with an increased deafness

> and that these noises were never pulsatile or carotid in origin and depended upon a particular state of the acoustic nerve and were not vascular in origin. This led me to believe that these symptoms, which were so serious and so worrying, resulted from a lesion of the special organ and were totally compatible with a state of good health...."

Prosper Ménière died on the 6th January 1862, aged 62, from pneumonia after being ill for only a few days. He was buried in the cemetery at Montparnasse outside Paris. Controversy persists over the correct spelling of his name. The family name was spelt Ménière, as on his tombstone but his writings were mostly under the spelling Menière. The latter spelling was used by his son Emile, who continued his father's work at the Imperial Institute for Deaf Mutes and, by his grandson Sergeant Jacques Menière, who was killed in the battle of the Somme, aged 38, in October 1916. Of all the controversies surrounding endolymphatic hydrops, this is surely the least worrying.

CHAPTER TWO

MEDICAL

MENIERE'S DISEASE

by

Jonathan Hazell FRCS

Consultant Neuro-Otologist to the R.N.I.D.

We now know that the condition is caused by an increase in the pressure of fluids in the inner ear (see The Ear and How it Works, R.N.I.D. publication). The cochlea (concerned with hearing) and semi-circular canals (concerned with balance) are bathed in this fluid which is called endolymph. Periodic increases in pressure of the endolymph (sometimes called endolymphatic hydrops) produce a dramatic disturbance of the hearing and balance at the same time. In addition to the giddiness, there is a loss of hearing in the affected ear, together with tinnitus which is generally low-pitched or rushing. After the attack, the hearing and tinnitus can improve and there may be long periods of time when the patient is entirely free of symptoms.

The disease is more common in men than in women. If the condition is untreated the hearing tends to become progressively worse, although in the early stages the hearing often returns to near normal levels. The hearing loss affects the low frequencies more than the high frequencies.

Although tinnitus can be a very distressing part of Ménière's Disease, particularly in the later stages, it is usually the vertigo and vomiting which trouble the majority of patients. The attacks are unpredictable and finding oneself lying on the floor in a public place, being sick, does not always bring out the most charitable feelings in other people.

Many patients with Ménière's disease are successfully diagnosed and treated by their general practitioner. Where possible, it helps to have some special tests performed to be quite certain that the diagnosis is correct. A pure tone audiogram is performed and this measures the hearing in each ear, at different frequencies. Many who have Ménière's disease suffer severe discomfort from loud sounds even though their hearing is impaired, and this feature (sometimes called recruitment) can be measured.

Investigation of the balance disorder can be quite complicated and take a long time. One test which is commonly performed is the caloric test. Each ear is gently irrigated with water, which is at a slightly different temperature from that of the body. This changes the temperature of the inner ear fluids, causing them to move in one or other direction. Examination of eye movements during this procedure can show how well the balance mechanism in each ear is working. In Ménière's disease there is often a reduction in the function of the affected ear on caloric testing. Many patients have an understandable fear of this investigation, as it might produce slight giddiness for a minute or so. However, it is an important investigation. It is not distressing if it is performed with care, and it yields important diagnostic information which can help greatly in the patients further management.

Management of Ménière's disease

Many forms of treatment are very effective, and may bring about long periods of freedom from the condition. After a while many patients cease to have disabling vertigo. As treatment may be needed over a long period of time, it is important to find a doctor with an interest in the condition, and heed the advice given about what may be a continuing programme of treatment and care.

Dietary Factors

Because there is an increase in fluid pressure in the inner

ear, most patients benefit from reducing salt intake which can cause fluid retention. Some specialists recommend keeping the general fluid intake down as much as possible, also steering clear of caffeine. Salt substitute can be obtained at chemists and used in cooking.

Medical Treatment

No two patients with Ménière's disease are alike and, as the frequency of attacks and course of the condition are very unpredictable, it is often hard to say whether the treatment is being effective. As there are often emotional factors at work, even the calm assurance of a competent practitioner sometimes produces periods of remission.

Serc (betahistine dihydrochloride) probably helps more Ménière's patients than any other drug, and is said to have a direct action on the blood circulation in the inner ear. Most patients with Ménière's disease will have tried it and it can be taken for long periods of time without ill-effect. Some patients who have severe attacks of vertigo need stronger anti-vertigo drugs such as Stemetil. It is often useful to have these available as a suppository because tablets may not be absorbed during an attack. There are a very large number of preparations, many of which may be helpful at one time or another, and successful treatment is often a matter of identifying the drug most helpful to the individual.

Hearing Loss

This usually affects only one ear and, while there is one normal ear, there may well be no difficulty in hearing in normal situations. In some patients, Ménière's disease may develop in the second ear. A trial of a suitable aid should always be offered to anyone with a hearing difficulty and, because of loudness discomfort or recruitment, this may need to incorporate a device for reducing the amplification of uncomfortable loud sounds. Excellent National Health hearing aids are available which incorporate these devices. Occasionally loudness discomfort is a serious problem and, where one ear is affected, a good fitting earplug (such as the EAR plug) may be helpful.

Tinnitus

Although tinnitus is not usually the most troublesome symptom, it is often relatively simple to treat in Ménière's disease. The tinnitus in Ménière's is very easily masked by a suitable tinnitus masker and, often, by a hearing aid alone. This is true when the tinnitus is of a low frequency or 'rushing' type; the high-pitched tonal tinnitus experienced by sufferers of Ménière's disease does not often respond as well and may not be the result of an increase in endolymph pressure. Patients with Ménière's disease whose vertigo responds to drug treatment may also experience a reduction in tinnitus; this is one of the few examples we have of successful treatment of tinnitus with tablets. However drugs such as Serc do not have any effect on the tinnitus (or vertigo) associated with conditions other than Ménière's disease.

Surgical Treatment

If all hearing has been lost in one ear and vertigo persists, a destructive operation can be performed down the ear canal (labyrinthectomy). This should not be contemplated when any useful hearing remains in the affected ear, in view of the possibility of second ear involvement. Other operations attempt to reduce the pressure of endolymph (e.g. drainage of the endolymphatic sac) or they may involve cutting the nerve of balance, where intractable vertigo persists. The endolymphatic sac is a small cul-de-sac coming from the inner ear, thought to be concerned with removal of its waste products. The drainage or decompression of this sac is often effective at controlling vertigo and sometimes results in an improvement in the hearing and tinnitus, at least in the short term.

QUESTIONS & ANSWERS

Questions frequently asked, answered by

Andrew Morrison FRCS

Chairman - Medical Advisory Committee

Part 1. Questions relating to the natural history and prognosis.

Q. How common is Ménière's disease? I seem to have met several people with this problem.

A. In the Caucasian population of Britain, Ménière's disease is quite common. It affects about one in every thousand of the adult population. It is principally a disease of middle age but it can start even in childhood, though not often in old age.

Q. Have you heard of any cases of children suffering from Ménière's disease?

A. It is unusual for Ménière's disease to start in childhood but it is nevertheless a well recognised problem. Most surgeons with large series of patients with Ménière's disease will have a number of childhood cases. There are many other cases of vertigo in childhood which have to be carefully excluded.

Q. I have had episodes of vertigo and dizziness on and off for many years but no hearing loss or head noises. Is this Ménière's disease?

A. There are many causes of vertigo, dizziness and instability. Ménière's disease is not usually diagnosed until the full triad of symptoms is present i.e. deafness, tinnitus and vertigo. Sometimes the deafness and tinnitus can precede the onset of the dizzy attacks by a number of years. It is very unusual for vertigo to start before the onset of deafness and tinnitus, though it probably does occur from time to time. In your case, however, with such a long history it is very unlikely that you have Ménière's disease.

Q. I have had Ménière's disease in my right ear for fifteen years but I am now experiencing head noises and a blocked feeling in the other ear. I am afraid this might be Ménière's disease. Can you advise me?

A. Unfortunately Ménière's disease becomes bilateral in up to fifty percent of patients with this disorder. Much depends upon the age of onset. The earlier the onset of the condition the more likely it is to become bilateral. If the condition remains unilateral for long periods of time, the chances of the second ear becoming involved diminish. In your case the symptoms are very suggestive and I think you should consult your doctor or specialist.

Q. My doctor tells me I have Ménière's disease but sometimes my hearing can be quite normal though I do get attacks of dizziness. Can you advise me?

A. In the early stages of Ménière's disease (which may continue for a number of years) fluctuation in hearing thresholds is a well recognised feature. Indeed it is almost the rule. Later in the disease, when the hearing loss becomes more severe, fluctuation is no longer a factor. I am sure your doctor is correct in his diagnosis.

Q. Is there a cure for Ménière's disease?

A. Regrettably, with the present state of our knowledge, we have no cure for this condition. Cures are sometimes recorded but it seems likely that these occur in patients who either did not have true Ménière's disease or alternatively, where the condition is so benign that very long periods of freedom occur.

Q. Has any relation between Migraine and Ménière's disease been established?

A. Association between the two conditions is well recognised and probably between 20% and 25% of patients with established Ménière's disease have a past history of Migraine. Not uncommonly, the Migraine started in childhood or adolescence and when it diminished in severity in middle age, Ménière's started. The ear problem need not be on the side of the usual Migraine, if indeed the Migraine is unilateral.

Q. I usually get warning of an attack but I understand that sometimes there is almost no warning. Is it safe to drive?

A. Fortunately the great majority of patients have adequate warning of an impending episode of vertigo and they can pull into the side of the road before the attack starts. In forty years experience of looking after some two thousand patients with this disorder, I can recall only one traffic accident which was due to a sudden attack of Ménière's disease. This frequency is so low that it must be lower than the National road traffic accident incidence. Having said that, there are a few patients who do have very severe episodes and drop attacks with no warning and in such patients it is wise to avoid driving when the condition is very active.

IMPORTANT NOTE FROM THE MENIERE'S SOCIETY

There are legal requirements for drivers who have Ménière's disease. Further information can be obtained from the Ménière's Society, enclosing an S.A.E., or write to the

D.V.L.C.This applies to the U.K. Sufferers in other countries are encouraged to contact their own local authorities.

Part 2. Questions on Causation

Q. I have recently developed Ménière's disease and my mother has the same condition. Is this hereditary?

A. Heredity plays a definite part in the aetiology of Ménière's disease. Most large series of patients who have been studied have revealed family incidence of between 3% and 8% first degree relatives with this condition. This is not strictly speaking a hereditary disease with a direct Mendelian inheritance. The chances of one of your own children having Ménière's disease are quite small.

Q. Can a fall cause Ménière's disease?

A. There is no direct proof that a fall will cause Ménière's disease. However, severe head injury, sufficient to cause concussion and temporary loss of consciousness, has been recorded as a possible predisposing factor in about 8% of patients with this disease. This is a much higher percentage of prior head injury than one would expect to find in the general population.

Q. My doctor tells me that my attacks of Ménière's disease are entirely related to stress and emotional factors. Do you agree?

A. I think there is little doubt that stress and severe emotional strain can help to precipitate episodes of Ménière's disease but they are not the cause of the problem. There have been numerous personality studies done on this condition, some of which have suggested personality type as a very important factor. Some studies, however, have usually been carried out during active phases of the disease. Similar studies should be performed when the condition is quiescent and an entirely different psychological profile would almost certainly emerge.

Q. Is any research into the cause of Ménière's disease being carried out in this country?

A. The cause of Ménière's disease is almost certainly multifactorial. Several things come together in the same patient. The most recent research in Britain is concentrated on the immunological aspects of the disease. It seems likely that in order to develop the condition the patient must have the correct hereditary background and probably belong to a specific tissue type. This tissue type may well make parts of the inner ear more susceptible to specific viral infections. Interesting research is progressing along these lines. If this proves to be correct, it should have very significant therapeutic implications.

Part 3. Questions on Surgical Treatment

Q. What operations are available for Ménière's disease? My doctor tells me that I am bound to lose the hearing if I have an operation.

A. There have in the past been a great many different surgical procedures employed, all with the intention of abolishing the attacks of dizziness. At present there are only three operations which are frequently employed in Britain and which carry a good prospect of controlling the symptoms.

Saccus Decompression

First is the surgery on the endolymphatic sac, part of the inner ear, but this is only effective in some 80% of patients and is normally only of value in the earlier stages of the disease. Patients for this surgery have to be very carefully selected. The results do not last for ever but many patients will go for years without trouble. This surgery preserves or improves the hearing with very little risk.

Neurectomy
The second operation, which is designed to abolish dizziness, involves dividing the vestibular nerve i.e. the nerve of balance, while leaving the nerve of hearing intact. This is a major procedure which is normally only performed in a small number of otoneurosurgical centres but it is very effective in abolishing attacks of vertigo. It is intended to maintain hearing.

Labyrinthectomy
The third operation, which is frequently performed, is that of labyrinthectomy when the balance part of the inner ear is surgically removed. This abolishes attacks of vertigo but it also causes total hearing loss in that ear. It does not affect the tinnitus as a rule, one way or another. It should be noted that some patients who have labyrinthectomy or vestibular neurectomy have post-operative imbalance which may take many months to disappear.

Q. I have severe Ménière's disease in one ear. I have seen a specialist who advises me to have a grommet inserted. Can you advise me?

A. There is no statistical or controlled evidence to show that the insertion of a grommet help patients with Ménière's disease. Sometimes, insertion of a grommet will make the condition worse.

There are many who believe that any treatment for this condition has a significant placebo effect. This is really the basis for the use of grommets. This implies that there is a major psychological factor in the aetiology of the disease which many of us do not accept.

Part 4. Questions relating to Medical Treatment

Q. Are diuretics of value in the treatment of Ménière's disease?

A. In Britain diuretics are not used extensively in the management of Ménière's disease though they are in the United States. Diuretics should only be taken under medical supervision. Some of them are ototoxic, that is, they can increase the damage to the ears. Others can damage the kidneys. The most commonly used - the thiazides - are probably the safest to use but they can give rise to disturbance of fluids and electrolytes in the body with loss of potassium. They also tend to precipitate diabetes. Some patients, however, appear to benefit from a short course of diuretics, especially females around the time of menses.

Q. Would a reduction in water intake mean no need to take tablets for this complaint?

A. Patients with Ménière's disease are frequently advised to reduce their salt and fluid intake but there are no controlled studies to verify the effect of this. Fluid should never be reduced to less than two pints daily. A strict salt free diet is very difficult to achieve and it is doubtful if the misery caused by such a diet is of great benefit.

Q. My doctor has prescribed Serc. He says I should take at least three tablets daily. Do you think this will cure my Ménière's disease?

A. Serc is a betahistine hydrochloride. It is a histamine

analogue and is one of the most commonly prescribed drugs for Ménière's disease, vertigo or dizziness, in this country. There have been a number of short trials to assess the efficacy of this drug and it does seem to be effective, at least for a period of time in some patients. Large double-blind studies have not been carried out. Histamine preparations such as this will aggravate symptoms of peptic ulceration so they are not indicated for people with dyspeptic symptoms. The usual recommended dose is two to four daily but occasionally larger doses can be tolerated.

Q. I have been taking three Stemetil tablets a day for over a year. Both my doctor and my chemist tell me that many people have been on this medicine for many years with no ill-effects. I would be worried about giving it up. Are there any ill-effects?

A. Stemetil is a phenathiazine. There are other drugs in the same category including Torecan. Such drugs are eliminated slowly from the body and taken over long periods, tend to accumulate. There is a risk of development of Parkinsonian symptoms such as rigidity and tremor. It seems likely that this problem is especially relevant in older age patients. The drug should be withdrawn if such symptoms develop. Stemetil, however, can be a useful drug during active episodes of vertigo. It can be given by injection, as a rectal suppository or orally as tablets. During acute spells, the sublingual preparation - trade name Buccastem - can be very helpful.

Q. I have been taking Stemetil for many years and my doctor has recently changed the treatment to Stugeron. Is this a good idea?

A. Stugeron has two pharmacological actions. It is a calcium antagonist though not a powerful one. This acts mainly on small blood vessels and prevents constriction of these vessels. In theory it therefore improves the micro circulation of the ear. At the same time it has a mild antihistaminic effect. This exemplifies the therapeutic dilemmas in managing Ménière's disease. Some patients will use the histamine analog and others use the antihistamine, each claiming some benefit! Stugeron, which is Cinnarizine, does seem the logical drug to use for this condition, though once again as with all medication, adequate controlled trials are lacking.

Q. My specialist told me that he had read something about the content from peanuts being investigated to help. Can this be explained please?

A. Peanuts are rich in nicotinic acid, one of the B vitamins. At one time, nicotinic acid, which is a powerful vasodilator, was used extensively in the management of Ménière's disease. It is still used occasionally with benefit during active phases. It does have the disadvantage of producing a rather unpleasant flushing of the head and face with pulsating headache in large dosages.

Q. Camomile tea seems to settle the pressure in my ears and help the vertigo. Is this possible?

A. The author has no experience of herbal medication. It is interesting, however, that Prosper Ménière himself was a great herbalist.

Q. Is oxygen of value in Ménière's disease?

A. In some clinics, Carbogen is used for the treatment of acute hearing loss and dizziness. This consists of the patient breathing in a mixture of oxygen and carbon dioxide. Some claim that it is of benefit in managing acute episodes but the value is doubtful.

Q. Does Ménière's disease have any effect on pregnancy?

A. During pregnancy some women find their Ménière's disease better and others worse. In theory, towards the end of pregnancy, fluid retention might aggravate the symptoms but this is purely theory. It is important, however, that drugs should not be taken during pregnancy, which might have a teratogenic effect.

Q. Can Ménière's disease patients wear hearing aids?

A. The hearing loss in Ménière's disease is sensory, that is it arises from damage to the cochlea rather than the nerve of hearing. Hearing aids can be of value to many patients with this condition provided they do not suffer from too much hyperacusis, that is loud noise causing intense discomfort. It is always worth having an assessment.

VERTIGO IN MENIERE'S DISEASE

by

Dr. Linda Luxon. BSc. FRCP

Consultant Physician in Neuro-Otology

> "......dizziness and ringing in the ears like all the bells of Halle, Leipzig, Erfust and Wittenberg. A foul fiend to whistle and roar in his ear and would cause disgusting attacks of nausea and make him so giddy that he would fall off his stool at work."
>
> Martin Luther (1483-1546)

In 1861, Prosper Ménière first described the clinical cluster of symptoms that soon became known as Ménière's disease. This condition is characterized by sudden, unexpected and recurring episodes of vertigo, which are associated with nausea and vomiting and occur simultaneously with difficulty in hearing and tinnitus. Ménière emphasized that the condition was associated with a disorder of the inner ear and not related to any disorder of the brain, as had been assumed previously.

It is helpful to define vertigo as an "illusion of movement". This may be subjective, in that the individual feels that he is moving, while the world is still; or objective, in that the world seems to move. There are many causes of vertigo, unrelated to Ménière's disease and it is a common mistake to assume that vertigo is synonymous with this disorder. A careful history together with a full assessment of vestibular function is often necessary to arrive at the correct diagnosis.

Under normal circumstances, information arises in each labyrinth and is carried to balancing centres within the brain. With the head in the resting upright position, the information from each ear is identical. When the head is tipped in one direction or another, there is an increase in the activity transmitted to the brain from one labyrinth, with an exactly similar decrease in activity from the opposite labyrinth (see diagram). In this situation, the brain "compares" the difference between the information coming from the two ears and can "judge" the precise direction and extent of any head movement. In this way, we know how our head is moving in space.

When disease alters the activity arising from one or other labyrinth, even in the resting position of the head, the information transmitted to the brain is different from the right and left ears. The brain "senses" this difference and incorrectly attributes it to a head movement, which the individual has not made. The brain thus misinterprets the balancing information and the subject experiences vertigo i.e. an illusion of movement. On the basis of this explanation, it is clear that any pathology which damages the balancing organs will give rise to a sensation of dizziness or vertigo.

In an attempt to clarify the diagnosis of Ménière's disease and provide clear guidelines, the Committee of the American Academy of Ophthalmology and Otolaryngology, chaired by Alford (1972) established criteria which should be used in the diagnosis of Ménière's disease. Three phases of the disease may be recognized. In the first early stage, the episodes of vertigo are associated with reversible fluctuating hearing loss, which commonly affects only the low frequencies of hearing. This stage is superseded by a period in which there is an established, but still fluctuating hearing loss, together with the episodes of dizziness. In the later stages of the disease, there is a non-fluctuating hearing loss upon which episodes of dizziness may be superimposed. Even at this late stage, patients will often complain of an increase in tinnitus or pressure in the ear immediately before, or during, their attacks of dizziness.

In general, patients with Ménière's disease find the vertigo so distressing that, particularly in the early stages, they may not notice the associated mild auditory symptoms. It is only as the vertigo subsides that the hearing loss and tinnitus may become obvious. Commonly the dizziness is associated with nausea and vomiting, together with pallor, sweating and slowing of the pulse rate. These symptoms are characteristic of any disturbance of balance and are familiar to everybody in association with motion sickness. Thus, it is clear that none of these symptoms are specific of Ménière's disease and merely reflect vestibular dysfunction. Although the vertigo of Ménière's disease may be severe as described above, many different forms may be seen and sometimes the vertigo may be relatively mild. By definition, it may last no more than 24 hours but may be of only 20 minutes duration. After it has subsided the patient may feel slightly off-balance and weak for the next 24 hours. The unpredictable nature of the attacks frequently leads to anxiety. The natural history of the disorder is that attacks tend to occur in clusters, which may last weeks or months, followed by periods of remission, during which there are no attacks. With the passage of time, the vertiginous attacks abate in severity and frequency, while the early fluctuant hearing loss becomes established.

Ménière's disease affects all age groups, but is not commonly seen in the third and fourth decades of life. The incidence in Great Britain is variously reported from 0.05 to 0.1% of the population. The occurrence appears to be determined by hereditary and environmental, rather than racial factors, but the precise aetiology remains obscure. It would seem that Ménière's disease is the late result of damage to the labyrinth, which may have passed unnoticed many years before the onset of symptoms. Pathological studies have identified that endolymphatic hydrops (too much fluid in the inner ear) is seen in patients with Ménière's disease, but the mechanisms precipitating this fluid excess are not clear.

A large number of clinical conditions enter into the differential diagnosis of vertigo, but a typical case of Ménière's disease can usually be identified quite readily. The therapeutic options in Ménière's disease are legion, but it must be recalled that a 60-80% success rate has been reported regardless of the treatment modality. The fluctuant nature of the disease and the high rate of placebo effect makes assessment of any treatment regime extremely difficult. As the precise cause of the disorder is unknown, by necessity treatment is symptomatic and encouraging results have been reported using a low sodium diet, vasodilator, antihistamines and a number of surgical procedures. However, only preparations Hydrochlorothiazide and Chlorthalidone have been convincingly demonstrated in double-blind crossover trials to improve symptomotology. There is no similar convincing data for other treatments which on an individual basis certain patients have reported as helpful, such as Prochlorperazine (Stemetil), Betahistine (Serc) and Cinnarizine (Stugeron). Various surgical procedures have been tried and would appear to be helpful in certain cases, but definite confirmation is lacking. Very rarely, in the face of severely disabling attacks of dizziness, destruction of the labyrinth or division of the vestibular nerve may be considered. Nonetheless, these procedures should be undertaken with the greatest caution, in view of the incidence of bilateral pathology in Ménière's disease.

DIAGRAM TO ILLUSTRATE CHANGES IN BALANCING ACTIVITIES WITH HEAD MOVEMENT.

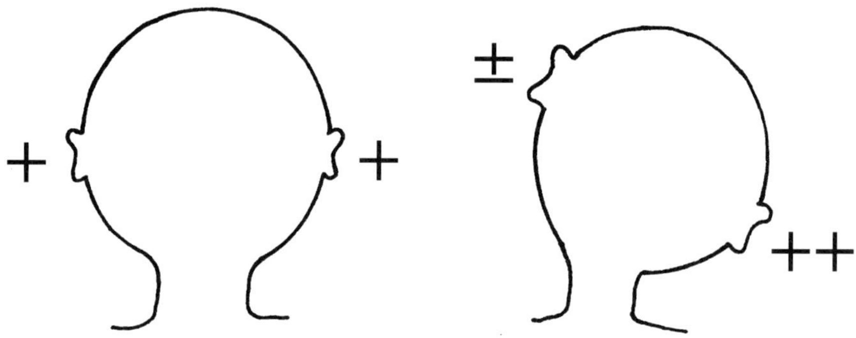

Resting position **Head tilt**

TINNITUS IN MENIERE'S DISEASE

by

Jonathan Hazell FRCS

Consultant Neuro-Otologist to the R.N.I.D.

Tinnitus is a symptom of a number of different conditions which can affect the ear or structure near the ear. In classical Ménière's Disease the tinnitus is very often associated with the attack of vertigo and fluctuating deafness. Very often it has a low pitched tonal quality, rather like an engine, or a dynamo running, or it may be of a hissing or rushing noise. Some people know that they are going to have an attack of vertigo because their tinnitus begins to get louder just before it. Whereas some Ménière's sufferers have no tinnitus in between attacks, others will have a background level, often of rushing tinnitus, which is continuous. In the majority of those experiencing Ménière's Disease, the tinnitus is not the most troublesome symptom. This is partly because the vertigo and vomiting may be a more serious complaint, or it may be that the tinnitus in Ménière's is not as severe as it is in certain other conditions. It is sometimes possible for the attacks of vertigo to lessen or disappear as time goes on and this may occur as a result or surgery or other medical treatment. In this case the tinnitus can sometimes become the most troubling symptom and requires separate management. It often responds remarkably well to symptomatic treatment with tinnitus maskers. Even though there may be quite a severe hearing loss in the affected ear, very low levels of masking often just make it inaudible. In other patients the correct fitting of a hearing aid to the ear, often using a vented mould, will not only improve hearing but will also help to mask tinnitus. Either or both of these solutions is worth trying if your tinnitus is troublesome, but remember that correct fitting of both a tinnitus masker or a hearing aid is essential and full counselling and instruction must be given.

Further information about all aspects of tinnitus may be obtained from:-

The RNID Tinnitus Help-Line
Unit 2
Pelham Court
Pelham Road
Nottingham
NG5 4AP
Tel: 0345 090210 (Voice/Minicom)

MENIERE'S DISEASE

Pressure appears to be a major factor in the destruction of vital areas of the inner ear - causing vertigo, tinnitus and deafness associated, singly or in combination, with Ménière's disease.

The following six photographs have been reproduced by kind permission of Duphar Laboratories Ltd., - the manufacturers of Serc.

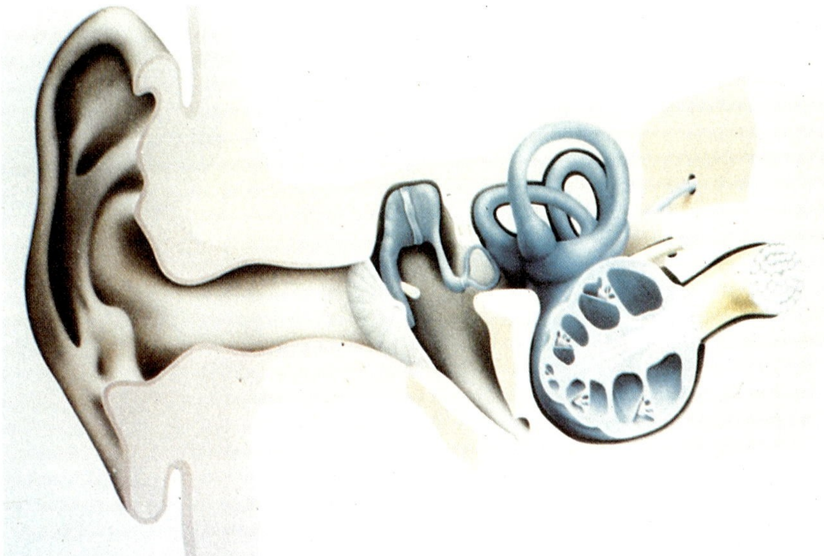

1. A stylised view of the ear, identifying the position of the inner ear which lies deep to the external auditory meatus and above the upper end of the Eustachian tube.

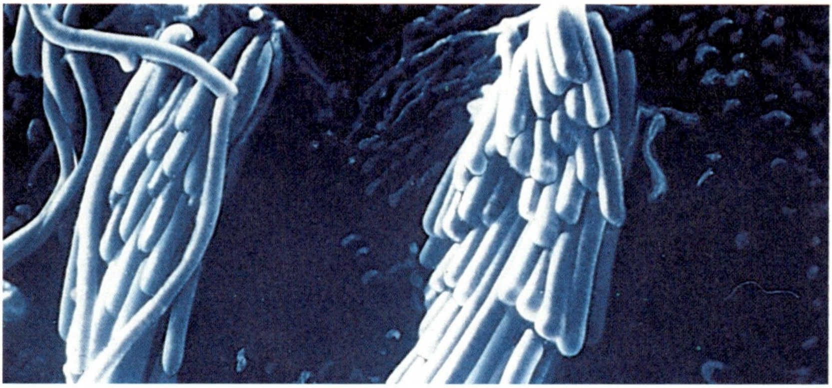

2. These are undamaged haircells. The haircells are situated at the expanded ends of the semi-circular canals. They are embedded in a gelatinous mass, the cupula, which floats in the endolymphatic fluid. Even slight rotations of the head cause the endolymph to move, which in turn moves the cupula. The resulting stimulation of the haircells signals information about the direction of rotation.

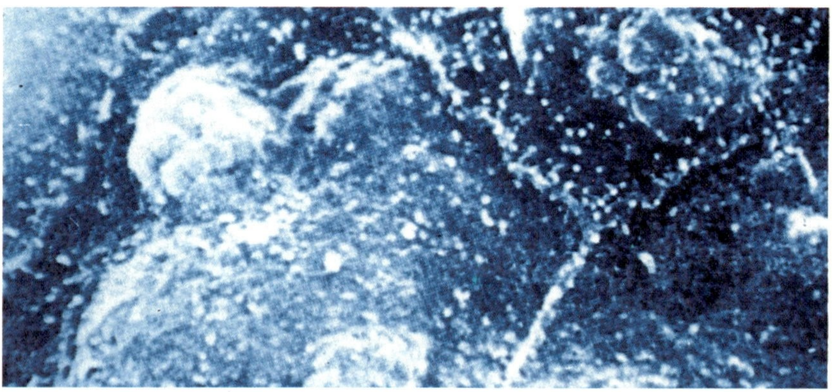

3. These are changed haircells, thought to have been damaged by pressure imbalance in the endolymph. All that is left are tiny stubs where the haircells once were.

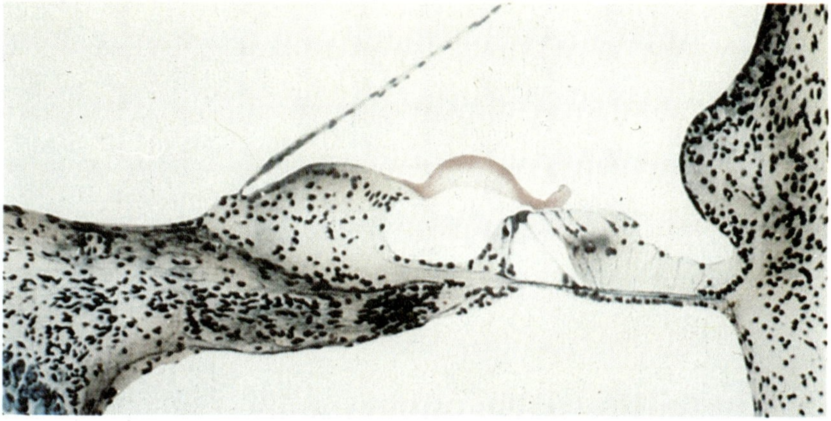

4. New visuals of Reissner's membrane, the membrane that separates the perilymph from the endolymph in the cochlea duct.

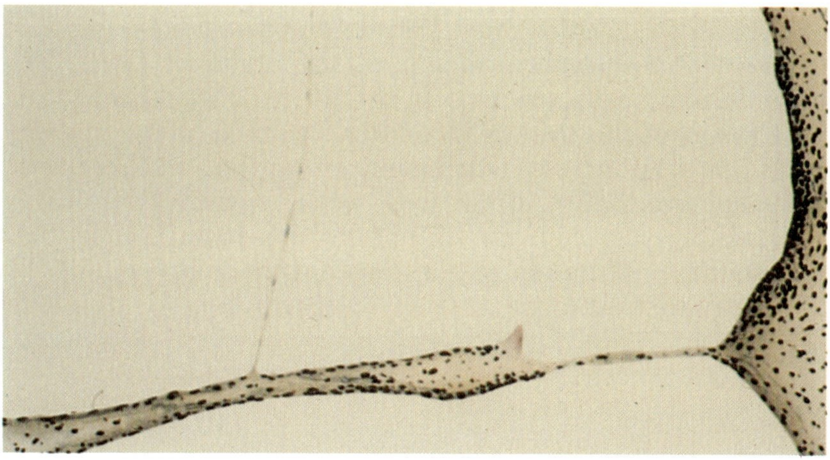

5. In Ménière's disease a pressure imbalance between the perilymph and endolymph causes the Reissner's membrane to shift due to distension. The consequent increase in pressure causes atrophy in the organ of Corti.

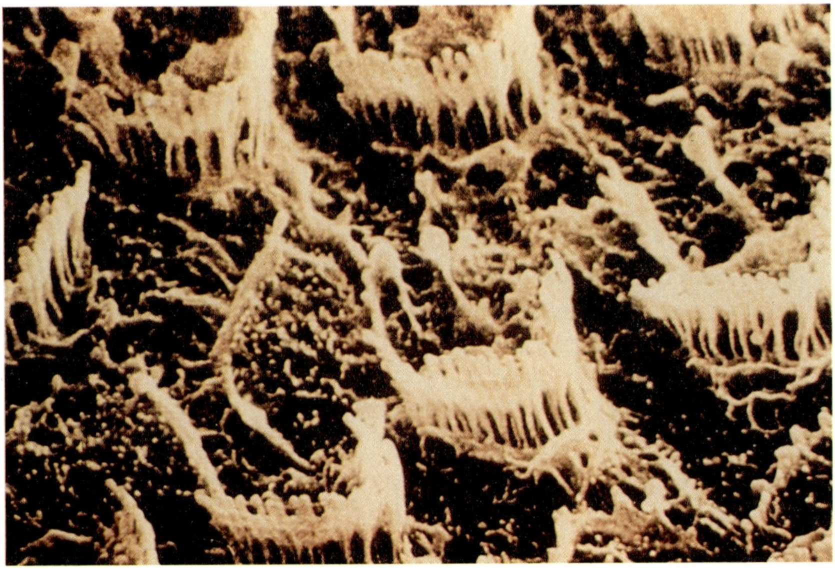

6. These are the auditory receptor cells found in the organ of Corti in the cochlea duct. Vibration of the endolymph duct causes sympathetic movement of the organ of Corti. The hairs of these cells are fixed in the reticular membrane, and as a result of the change in relative position of the cellbody to its hairs, an impulse is transmitted via the auditory nerve. Hearing gradually diminishes with ageing - probably because receptor cells die off one by one. It is thought that a similar, but more rapid degeneration is caused by Ménière's disease.

In the many letters we receive from sufferers, we realised that very few had been encouraged to try the following exercises to help relieve their vertigo. These exercises are well known generally but because of possible underlying factors, it is essential to obtain your doctors recommendations before embarking on this régime.

The Society should also point out, there are limitations to the use of vestibular head exercises for patients with Ménière's disease. These type of exercises are of greatest value in the rehabilitation after labyrinthectomy or vestibular nerve section.

CAWTHORNE-COOKSEY EXERCISES

INTRODUCTION

The balance parts of the two ears complement each other, sending equal impulses to the brain which are essential for the maintenance of equilibrium of the head and body.

If either or both centres are damaged, equilibrium is upset. The result of this is vertigo or giddiness which may be accompanied by nausea and vomiting. Although this condition may be very frightening, it is not serious in that it does not, in itself, threaten life. It can, furthermore, be overcome by carrying out special exercises.

The purpose of these exercises is to build up a tolerance mechanism in the brain which compensates for the unequal balance of the two ears. The exercises stimulate the development of this tolerance mechanism and the more diligently and regularly they are performed, the sooner will vertigo disappear.

The exercises should be carried out persistently for at least five minutes, three times a day and for as long as vertigo persists. This could be for up to three months. A conscious effort should be made to seek out the positions and movements that cause vertigo in so far as can be tolerated because the more frequently vertigo is induced, the more quickly is the brain compensation mechanism built up.

Certain medications help to control the vertigo while brain compensation is achieved and any such tablets should be taken regularly during the course of exercises.

Meanwhile, as normal a life as possible is recommended. Early return to work and recreation are helpful in rehabilitation.

Diligence and perseverance will be required but the earlier and more regularly the balance exercise régime is carried out, the faster and more complete will be recovery to normal activity.

The exercises follow:-

A. In Bed

1. Eye movements - at first slowly, then quickly.
   a) up and down
   b) from side to side
   c) focusing on finger moving from 3 feet to 1 foot away from the face.

2. Head movements - at first slowly, then quickly. Later with eyes closed.
   a) bending forwards and backwards
   b) turning from side to side.

B. Sitting

1. As A. 1 and 2.

2. Shoulder shrugging and circling.

3. Bending forwards and picking up objects from the ground.

C. Standing

1. As A. 1 to 2 and B. 1 to 3.

2. Changing from sitting to standing position with eyes open and then shut.

3. Throwing a small ball from hand to hand (above eye level).

4. Throwing a small ball from hand to hand (under the knee).

5. Change from sitting to standing and turning around in between.

D. Moving About (recommended group activity)

1. Circle around centre person who will throw a large ball and to whom it will be returned.

2. Walk across the room with eyes open and then closed.

3. Walk up and down a slope with eyes open and then closed.

4. Walk up and down steps with eyes open and then closed.

5. Any game involving stooping or stretching and aiming such as skittles, bowls or basket ball.

DIETARY FACTORS

Whilst debatable, dietary factors have to be considered in the effective treatment of Ménière's disease. The diversity of the condition, coupled with individuality, necessitates talking in general terms rather than quoting hard and fast rules. Having said this, there exists a standard list of rules that sufferers should be aware of and try to comply with. Although some have raised question about their effectiveness, most make sense in improving ones general health. In all of the following, at least a reduction is recommended:-

Salt
Use salt substitute as an alternative.

Fluid
Remember that a human being requires an intake of at least 2 pints of fluid per day to maintain life. The total includes the fluids within food consumed during the day.

Caffeine
Please note that caffeine is in tea and coffee, as well as many other products such as chocolate and some well known soft drinks. Also note that decaffeinated products are not necessarily caffeine free.

Alcohol
Increased levels in tinnitus often reported especially with red wine. It is also unwise to mix medication and alcohol.

Smoking
Reported to have similar effect on tinnitus and bad for the health anyway.

Stress
Avoid at any cost or at least "manage" unavoidable stress. Rest and relaxation of great value.

(It must be said here that some sufferers have reported no ill effects from consuming any one of the previously mentioned substances. This underlines the diversity of the condition.)

Further Suggestions

It is virtually impossible to avoid salt completely because it is not always declared as an ingredient in prepared food. If salt must be used, use it in cooking but not on the table.

Possible "salty food" to avoid:- ham, bacon, salt beef, tinned meat, salty tinned fish, products in brine, sardines, smoked haddock and kippers; sea foods such as shrimps, cockles, winkles and mussels.

Other products having high salt content are stock cubes and beef, yeast and vegetable spreads. A surprising amount of salt is in cheese, tomato ketchup and baked beans.

Suggested Alternative Flavourings

Unsalted nuts, sugar, jam, marmalade, herbs, spices. Fruits such as lemons, apples and oranges (although citrus fruits have been mentioned as aggravating the condition on more than one occasion). Vegetables such as mushrooms, onions, red/green/yellow peppers (not the hot ones) and tomatoes.

Please note this is not a lesson in cookery or a suggestion that you reduce your meals to an occasion to be dreaded. Experiment and if you find palatable foods which do not aggravate your condition, so much the better (the editors themselves enjoy many of the foods on the 'hit list' to no ill effect). A reduction in salt will at least give your taste buds a chance to inform you of the real flavour of food.

APPROXIMATE SALT CONTENT

Product	per/oz	mg/salt
Milk	-	14.0
Cheese	-	173.0
Cream Cheese	-	85.0
Cottage Cheese	-	128.0
Natural Yoghurt	-	22.0
Eggs	-	40.0
Honey	-	3.0
Beef	-	16.0
Pork	-	18.0
Bacon	-	420.0
Tinned Ham	-	355.0
Chicken	-	23.0
Liver	-	26.0
Kidney	-	57.0
Fresh Haddock	-	36.0
Herring	-	19.0
Kipper	-	281.0
Butter	-	247.0
Unsalted Butter	-	2.0
Margarine	-	227.0
Potatoes	-	2.0
Brussel Sprouts	-	1.0
Cauliflower	-	2.0
Fresh Peas	-	0.3
Frozen Peas	-	0.9
Tinned Peas	-	65.0
Mushroom	-	3.0
Oranges	-	1.0
Tinned Peaches	-	0.3
Dried Prunes	-	4.0
Cornflakes	-	298.0
Instant Coffee	-	10.0
Yeast Extract	-	1318.0

Milk Chocolate	-	78.0
White Bread	-	153.0
Wholemeal Bread	-	153.0
Smoked Ham	-	719.0
Tinned Crab	-	156.0
Tinned Salmon	-	153.0
Salami	-	358.0
Corned Beef	-	1221.0
Natural Peanut Butter	-	1.0
Salted Peanut Butter	-	199.0
Yeast (comprised baler)	-	4.5
Yeast (dried brewers)	-	34.0

THE CONSULTATION

by

Mrs. Barbara Parkinson.

Poynton, Cheshire.

Have you ever come out of the consulting room and realised that you have made a complete hash of the visit?

Well here are a few tips.

There are three things to consider before you go to the appointment.

1. Arrange to take a friend or relative with you. This is most important if you have a hearing problem. No doctor will mind someone sitting in on the consultation.
2. Write a list of questions you wish to ask and do not be frightened to use it.
3. Leave yourself plenty of time to get to the appointment. Arriving flustered will not help in any way.

If you go on your own, ensure that the receptionist knows you are hearing impaired. When your name is called out, you might not hear it.

When you are called for your consultation, remember the doctor is not God - beneath that white coat beats the heart of a normal human being who may not be feeling well themselves that day.

Keep to the facts and try not to waffle or get sidetracked - remember that you are probably not the only Ménière's sufferer they will see that day.

If the doctor says something you do not understand, interrupt and ask for the information to be repeated in simpler terms. If tests are suggested, ask what they are and what to expect. Remember that it is your body and you do not have to agree to anything you are not 100% happy about. If a course of tablets are suggested, ask for clear instructions on how many, how often and for how long should they be taken. Ask about any side effects and if you think you are unable to remember any of the instructions, ask for them to be written down.

If you try to follow this plan, my experience shows that I am happy and, hopefully the doctor is happy, when saying "goodbye" to a satisfied customer.

Don't forget to make another appointment before you leave, if this has been suggested.

Good Luck!

'COPING WITH MENIERE'S A PSYCHOLOGICAL ASPECT'

by

Mrs. C.B.

Maidstone, Kent.

Ménière's is not the worst that can happen to you. It's not fatal, and most of the time you feel normal. But when it strikes, it really strikes! You are helpless for the duration. It is unpredictable and incurable and is bound to change your life.

How, and how much, it changes your life depends a lot on the frequency and severity of the attacks. Some people cope well with amazingly bad situations, others go to pieces easily. You can teach yourself to be more like the first group.

The actual attacks are a medical matter. In time you will find out just how far your attacks can be controlled. Then knowing the bottom line of just what you've got to put up with, you can take positive steps to cope with it.

The worst hours are actually when you are under attack. Your body has no choice but to sweat it out, but your mind can help you through. You don't have to dwell on the benefits of euthanasia, you can think positive thoughts. "This will stop. It always stops. It's mucked up today, but only today. When it stops, I can ...." and imagine yourself doing whatever you like doing. This is called "coping self-talk" and is tailor made, by you, to suit you.

Afterwards it is easy to fall into the self-doubt trap, something keeps happening that is out of your control. An attack may strike any time, anywhere, no matter who you are with or how busy you are. When you're in a phase of attacks it can happen every day or more. You may need a lot of looking after. This can make you feel useless. Sometimes the people around you may exacerbate this feeling because they do not realise how disabling it is. They may think you should "pull yourself together". There is little point in expressing anger to those people, anger begets more anger and leads to pointless rows. Instead you can extend your 'coping self-talk' to assertive talk to others. Give them facts. You have Ménière's. You are intermittently utterly disabled. It is extremely inconvenient, always to yourself, and sometimes to others as well, but it has to be tolerated as and when it happens. The cause is wholly physical, the result of an imbalance of fluids in your ear. You can neither consciously nor subconsciously bring it on, nor can you put a stop to it or obviously you would. In between attacks you are as capable as you ever were. Don't let having Ménière's make you feel that in any way you are a lesser person.

When you have an attack amongst strangers, it is probable that none of them will have ever heard of Ménière's, and you won't feel like in-depth discussion. The Ménière's Society SOS card helps in this situation, with its graphic description of symptoms. If you have this card and are in a fit state, produce it. With your name and address on it it asks that they help you get home and not be taken to hospital. If you don't have the card with you, devise a few short sentences you can use, like, "It's my ears, they swell up inside and I can't balance till they go down again. It's not as serious as it looks, please help me get home". If you've rehearsed what to say beforehand it is easier not to panic.

The repeated sudden immobilisation will prevent you from doing many things that you want and need to do, and this will affect many people in your circle, particularly your family who may be worried and upset. It can be helpful to pose the question:- “What’s the worst that could happen?”. This is double barrelled. If the worst is not too bad you can come to terms with it, and if the worst is very bad you can take avoiding action. For example, if your worst fear is that you will have an attack just after you’ve put the chip pan on, and that the house will burn to the ground with you inside it, then you can use oven chips. The worst that can happen then is that the chips will be burnt to a frazzle. If however, your worst fear is that you’ll look a fool in front of strangers, does that really matter? If strangers are so unkind as to think you foolish for being ill, is their good opinion worth having?

You can involve your family in this. If they feel perturbed, they too can think about the worst possible outcome and either come to terms with it or take preventative measures. Then they can remind you of this and of any other coping strategy you’ve found helpful, whenever you’re too down to think straight - and possibly vice versa.

It is well worthwhile to find time to talk through all the aspects of your Ménière’s with your family. Talking is part of the process of coming to terms with it, but don’t let the discussions turn into ever more horrific speculations about what could happen. Get hold of the facts so you know what to expect. Even small children should be told at a level they can understand. Being told “everything is all right” when it clearly isn’t will confuse and frighten them. Being told “Daddy will keep getting ill like this but he will always get better again” will enable them to adjust. Once everyone knows what is likely to happen you can decide together what to do about it, both in practical terms, and in terms of giving each other support.

“What makes things easier for your family?”. There are as many ways of coping as there are families, so work out your best way. Although you cannot be cured, at least not yet, you can use psychology to get you through and help you keep it in perspective. It is a nasty, horrible, boring, tyrannical nuisance, but not a tragedy. You can learn to live with it and live happily.

NB. The writer is a Ménière's Society member and has a degree in psychology. Her husband is a counselling psychologist.

CHAPTER THREE

'MY STORY'

'NO, NO, HE ISN'T DRUNK, REALLY'

by

Mrs. M.N.

Loughborough, Leics.

I don't know if they believed me, those three kind people in the space of 100 yards who offered to help as I was walking with my husband, trying to stop him from crashing through Woolworth's large glass doors which he was listing threateningly towards.

It was one of his more sudden attacks, triggered by trying on a pair of shoes and bending to fasten them. We made a rapid ahead-of-schedule departure from the shoe shop, leaving the assistant wondering what she had done wrong. I did return later to get the shoes.

That particular attack was frightening by its suddenness and for a while he wouldn't venture forth on his own. Touch wood, attacks like that have eased a lot now, and we can pause for a while and look back and remember the time ....

.... our Italian guide, Luigi, had to leap into action for us in a sea-front café in Amalfi. Whilst his spaghetti bolognese got cold and ours went completely to waste, Luigi got the waiters organised 'pronto' to provide a make-shift bed in an unused room. After half an hours lie-down, my husband had to be better, whether-or-no, as the 'unused' room began to fill with another coach party. We were lucky that time as a gentle walk round got him at least mobile, though he still felt dreadful. However, the sensational scenery on the next part of our journey from Amalfi to Ravello helped to get him out of it - a little.

.... as we were going by cable-car up the almost sheer mountain side, all 7000ft of it, from Palm Springs desert floor, to the greenly wooded mountain top. Going over the cable-car points was enough to jolt him and trigger the dreaded big M. So at the top we had a nice cool drink, a long sit down, took our photos and got down again as best we could - back to the 100 degree heat - don't ever go there in July!

.... as we had our farewell party. Leaving Australia at the end of a three week stay, our Philippino sister-in-law had arranged a leaving party for us, invited all her compatriots (there are lots of them around Sydney) and organised a super disco with flashing lights. We-e-ell, we had to stay in a quiet room well away from the party action, looking like party-poopers. (Yes, we have travelled around a bit. That is in case the illness goes from bad to worse and we won't be able to travel at all).

He has got, over the years, very good at disguising his attacks unless they are really severe. Long practice at having to keep on working, hanging on to the nearest surface with one hand while carrying on a conversation with someone, and avoiding having to cross open spaces. Sometimes when he has had to work late, close colleagues have been warned that if they find him lying under the desk to just leave him there.

Some of his worst attacks though have been abroad when away on business, usually alone, at night, in strange surroundings, - not at all fun.

It can be very worrying being the on-looker, you feel the weight of responsibility for doing something when an attack strikes, which usually occur in the worst circumstances. I have described some of our more colourful occasions, but there have been others which were very grim, and irreplaceable events ruined, - the family all together for the first time in years and where's Dad? - Upstairs having one of his attacks.

However, people can be very kind and you certainly find your real friends.

I do find my local Ménière's Group as useful for myself as my husband, it welcomes the "helpers", and they too understand more from meeting other sufferers. We have all gained a sense of companionship and solidarity as well as having a good laugh - possibly the best medicine of all.

'MY MENIERE'S DISEASE'

by

Mr. R.B.

Cambridge

In the early summer of 1967 I was driving an old Ford Escort van along Mill Road, Cambridge, when I felt a bit dizzy, something that had happened several times on and off over the previous dozen years or so and which I had ascribed to the after effects of rheumatic fever during National Service. This time it lasted a bit longer. I had to stop the car; I had a splitting headache and a pounding in the ears. Left with a Systolic murmur, which sounds serious enough to keep a straight face about, and a 30% disability army pension (which H.M.G. doesn't dispense without due cause), I assumed I must be suffering a sort of heart attack, stroke or boiling blood pressure - my greatest concern was how to cause the least embarrassment and get myself home.

By screwing up my eyes, concentrating exceptionally hard and driving dangerously slowly, I got home. Staggered up the stairs and into bed, feeling like a landlubber in a sinking ship. I was not drunk, had no pain in the chest, it couldn't be a heart attack or angina but the world kept going round and round every time I closed my eyes.

"I think you've got Ménière's disease", opined the friendly GP, who was finally summoned, his advice being to prop myself up in the corner of the room and to move my head very slowly, if at all.

After a fortnight, I had stopped reeling and being sick and could stand straight enough to be led gently by a kindly wife to the Ear, Nose and Throat department of the nearest hospital, where a cheery consultant confirmed that I had gone partially deaf in one ear. I had noticed.

"Sorry about that, old boy. It may come back, but generally the hearing gets worse and worse until the nerve in the inner ear finally burns out and you go stone deaf. Good news is, though, the other symptoms disappear, and you've always got the other ear. Nature's kind.

"Thank you doctor". I appreciated his homely philosophy. "Is there anything I can do about it?"

"Next to nothing, old chap. We've only known about it for a hundred years. Fighter pilots in the war seemed to get it quite a lot. Your ear-drums look a bit scarred."

"Yes, I've done a bit of flying and high-diving."

"Well, that's it, then. Oh, give up salt, by the way. They say it helps, and cut down on your liquids - say, no more than a pint and a half a day."

"You mean beer."

"No - in all, total everything."

"Really, why?"

"They say it helps."

I eventually returned to work as a teacher, got used to recognising the symptoms of an attack on the way; the stab in the head, the electric switch across the brain and the rising nausea in the chest. Sit down, grip the desk, smile at the class and hope for the best. Mind over matter. The temperature goes up, the mouth dries up like a wind in the desert, and then, with luck it passes, but you dare not get up for a while when the bell goes for fear that the floor won't be there when you put your foot down.

You get used to swivelling your good ear towards the sounds you need to pick up, but you can't avoid giving offence at a dinner party to the lady on your dead side who thinks you're cutting her because she's plain or just not interesting. There's nothing wrong with me, she thinks, and concentrates on the bloke on the other side. She's guessed, I reckon, I'll have to explain. "I'm afraid I'm deaf in this ear", you may say cheerily. Just my luck to get sat next to an invalid, she smiles. And the tinnitus bashes on, now like a drum roll, now like a jet engine, pulsing and whining, never, never giving up. What to do with your bloody head? Thank God for the loud noises at parties, when nobody expects to hear what anybody's saying and the demon noise inside the head is battered into insignificance by the row without, and, if you reel as you walk, people just think you're drunk, so never mind.

"Look. old boy," said the friendly GP the next year I saw him. "They're trying out a new treatment, simple operation, all over in a day".

"Oh yes," I said suspiciously, despondently.

Never let them cut you up, my old father used to advise, believing he had lost a vital organ he could ill spare when under anaesthetic.

"It's called a grommet."

"Sounds evil," I responded.

"Worth a try, nothing to lose."

Three days before Christmas 1968, I was put on a slab. What an absolutely glorious feeling it is when that needle begins to take effect, the floating loveliness of sinking into Xanadu, courtesy of the National Health. However, when you come round, you pay for it by having to spend a night on a plank bed in the public ward with the lights left on. Anyway, home in time for Christmas with a grommet neatly inserted through the ear drum in order, so the theory goes, to let the air out of the middle ear and thus release pressure. Now, I think there's quite a lot in the pressure theory. I know that when I'm abroad in a warm climate on holiday and the barometer is up, I feel fine, while back in the cold and damp of my native fens, I feel abysmal. What about the South of France on NHS prescription for the Ménière's fraternity? After all, it's a bloody French disease, isn't it?

So we sit down to our 1968 Christmas dinner, and father with his new ear piece, which, however, encouragingly, was helping the hearing not a little. (Mind over matter again?) "Don't ask me how it works, old boy. We just tried it out and it seemed to do the trick for some, if not all." So it works. Who cares if magic is irrational?

Happy family circle, old-fashioned father at the head of the table with carving knife and fork in front of the steaming turkey that mother has carefully cooked. Lift the knife and bang! What's happened? Has the turkey exploded. No, not at all. Father has tipped upside down - after only one small dry sherry before lunch - can't regain his balance and the three-year old is picking a little pink tubey thing off the floor on the other side of the room. "What's this, mummy?" It's daddy's grommet, which had shot across the room like a bullet out of father's ear-hole. Perhaps it's something to do with all the cannons firing and the church bells pealing away in double time. Patient and long-suffering wife helps grommet-less husband back up to bed, where he enjoys the rest of the holiday.

"No thanks, old man, I don't think I'll bother about another grommet in the ear."

Sixteen years pass by - how time flies when you're having a good time! And I was having a good time. Children growing up, business doing fine, Ménière's laying dormant. Still rather deaf and had to watch it a bit, though, but nothing I can't manage. Not yet. Then, in the summer of 1984, I begin to get more regular attacks; I have some tinnitus in my other ear, too. Pray God, no. They said it's a million to one chance getting the bloody cursed thing in both ears. Don't panic. Go to new friendly GP, the old one having had to take early retirement due to over-work and a lifetime of bearing witness to the ineffable frailties of the human situation. His replacement was away on a beano at an American university, lecturing to undergraduates on the useful effects eating slugs may have on the advances of senile dementia. I was seen by a female locum. "Probably a bit of wax in the old eustachian, I reckon," she judged matily. It sounded rude. I declined a washout politely. "I have Ménière's disease," I explained. "Oh yes," she said, as if it was somewhere to go for your holidays.

So back to the experts at the new hospital. My goodness me, they have come a long way in all these years, gleaming spectroscopes, lobotomy probes, scanners and spanners and all sorts of excellence and brilliance - and the hearing measuring electronic devices. Who says the NHS doesn't know how to spend money? Gadgets galore.

"Look, old boy. I'm awfully sorry to tell you this, but it's Ménière's in the other ear."

"Yes, I had noticed."

"The tests confirm."

"So, all that to prove I'm now deaf in both ears."

"Not quite that, there's the good news. And I don't pretend to understand."

Strange, isn't it, the way the medical lexicography doesn't alter with time and how the knowledge seems to be much the same. When I was a young teacher, we had a blackboard and chalk, and forty-five pupils in a class and now they've got ..... but that's another story.

"OK. What is it?"

"Well, your other ear still has 25% hearing, so that when this one goes - if it does, that is, because, mind, it's up and down and sometimes it comes back for a long time."

"Why?"

"Well we don't know, really; it's something to do with sodium and potassium salts crossing the membranes in the inner ear. But we're pretty ignorant about what goes on at the cell level."

"Is no one doing any research on it?"

"No money, I'm afraid, and it's not a popular illness, is it now? Not like cancer which everybody knows about and raises money for."

I supposed it wasn't and I looked around the surgery at the ten million pounds worth of machines and I wondered about consultant's salaries and grommets and measuring machines.

"Don't you think it's worth finding out what it's all about before you go in for all this lot?"

He gave me a hard look and probably regretted having been so frank. His professional manner returned.

"Well now. I can get you a hearing aid for the 25% ear. It will probably take a bit of getting used to. It'll set up a few inner vibrations and electrical currents that might upset you. But it's worth a try."

"I look forward to it," I said happily.

"It's marvellous the way that ear's burnt out the Ménière's and left you so much hearing. Usually you go stone deaf."

"There's still time," I said. "Don't despair."

'TERRY'

by

A friend

Terry was diagnosed as having Ménière's disease in 1983 at the age of 39. Explaining that he had experienced these symptoms since the age of 18 and after looking at his medical history, the doctors at the hospital agreed that it had probably gone "undiagnosed" all these years, although, except for the tinnitus and very gradual hearing loss, the vertigo attacks did go into remission for many years.

The recent attacks started with two or three every week for varying periods, usually starting in the early morning. His own GP on maternity leave, the locum immediately recognised it as Ménière's disease and made an appointment for him to see the Ear, Nose & Throat Specialist at the local hospital. After the usual tests, the diagnosis was confirmed.

After the initial shock and not really 'taking it all in', Terry's thirst for knowledge on this condition unknowingly was about to change his whole life. Pressurising the doctors for full details, stopping and questioning the doctors when they said something he didn't quite understand. Eventually the picture unfolded with basic details on dietary factors, possible operations, trials with a variety of medication and finally the knowledge and acceptance that 'there is no cure'.

From this time onwards Terry's problems increased. His present job as Senior Playleader on an Adventure Playground became an impossibility through safety factors. On applying for another job and being accepted, he asked his GP if stress was an aggravating factor in this condition. He was assured that it was not and on that advice, accepted the job. It was working with young offenders, trying to get them working experience in the public sector! This obviously proved too much for him and after nine months, his Hearing Therapist felt it was time for him to quit, saying that he was definitely too ill to work. After talking to his doctors, they all agreed that Terry would probably never work again.

For a long time Terry could not accept his Ménière's and tried a variety of medication with little advice on any of them including any possible side effects. As time went on Terry lost confidence in any treatment suggested to him. He felt that his own GP.'s did not understand how much this condition was affecting him personally and posed these questions:-

"Is it because doctors know little about this condition and tend to make light of it?"

"Is it fear (considering the first question) because they do not know the answers to questions suffers might ask?"

"Is it because they do not have the time to counsel properly?"

"Is it the old adage that they see an 'ailment' coming through the surgery door and not a human being?"

Social life began an inevitable downward spiral. Friends seemed to lose contact because, never sure when an attack would come, Terry declined invitations to socialise rather than let people down.

Unemployment and its stigma brought depression through a variety of experiences. He felt labelled because he appeared to be a 'risk' to employers. One Christmas, with pressures from his children (and wanting one himself), Maureen (his wife) and himself decided to buy a video recorder. Hire purchase being the only way possible, after completing the form, the shop assistant said he would have to check with head office as Terry was unemployed. They refused the deal because of 'lack of credibility'. Terry was shattered. In anger and to avoid disappointing their children and pushing their funds to the limit, they eventually bought one for cash. Financial hardship inevitably followed and they decide that Maureen would have to be the main "wage earner", Terry taking over the role at home and looking after the children. The children's attitude to Dad also seemed to alter, looking more to Mum as the decision-maker. This role reversal affected his perception of his status in life and his depression deepened. Even as a young man he had always held posts of responsibility in employment, this situation was becoming unbearable. He lost confidence in himself and from being a confident, outgoing person, for a time, he avoided all situations where new experiences arose or where there were fresh people to be met.

He became frustrated at trying to explain the reasons why he could not hold a permanent job to people who seemed to disbelieve he had a handicap. Everything became a hard and lonely fight and with little advice and support forthcoming he began to lose all direction in life.

After seeing a Disablement Resettlement Officer at the local Job Centre, he was told that his best course of action was to go to a Rehabilitation Centre. Having already experienced one some years earlier when he had an accident in the motor trade and found he could no longer work on cars due to a severe back injury, he declined the offer. The experience was so traumatic, he did not want a repeat performance. Because one is not usually given the option of going, but usually told to go "or loose your benefits", Terry lived in fear of being "sent back" - this stress adding to his problems.

Although he eventually qualified for Invalidity Benefit, the regular medical's required became something to be feared. It was clear to Terry that the doctor carrying out the medical had little knowledge of the condition and he was regularly declared fit for work. This started a "Merry-Go-Round" (to use Terry's own words) because, if he was successful in getting an interview, application forms all seemed to gear their questions towards "do you experience giddy spells ?" By the time he had explained what Ménière's disease was, he realised he had just talked himself out of a job. Eventually the Job Centre would say "You are not fit for work!" and he would be back on sick leave, and so the Merry-Go-Round would continue. He remembers one doctor he saw at a medical telling him "well don't tell your prospective employer that you have the condition!" As this is highly illegal, Terry wisely did not take this advice.

When it was clear that the relationship between himself and his GP. had deteriorated through disagreements on his condition, Terry decided to look for another practice. This was not without its difficulties and brought added strain when at one point his entire family were without any medical support, Terry taking responsibility for this eventuality. Explaining his situation to the local Family Practitioners Committee, they quickly took up his case and found another practice who, with the reservation that they discuss the matter, were willing to include his family on their books. Explaining fully the situation Terry found himself in, they were happy to include his entire family in their practice. He is still with them now and is very happy with the support and interest he had for so long desperately needed.

Maureen supported him throughout and his saviour was his Hearing Therapist. Her constant support and ready accessibility was a valuable 'bolt hole' he could go to. When Maureen became confused about Terry's behaviour, the therapist spent valuable time talking to Maureen, helping her to understand Terry's fears.

With growing understanding and confidence, Terry started voluntary work at the local school, providing assistance in reading skills to the children and helping out with special events. He helped on their weekly visits to the swimming pool and assisted with any day visits. He also joined the scouts, becoming the local scout leader. At about this time, his Hearing Therapist had heard of a woman who had appealed on the 'See Hear' programme on television for a response to her idea of a self help group for sufferers. Unable to make the first meeting because of an attack, Terry attended the second and it became clear that this was his niche in life. In fact it became a life saver to him. With support from his wife and Marie (Founder of the Society), coupled with guidance, it helped to restore his credibility and gave him a chance to help others.

The support group became the Ménière's Society, gaining charitable status and expanded rapidly. Terry is now fully employed by the Society as Co-Ordinator at the Woking based office. Unfortunately his other voluntary work had to stop but he still keeps in touch with occasional visits. He is also involved in teaching camping skills, something he has done for many years.

In 1984 it was found that Terry had bilateral Ménière's (both ears). Life continues to be a struggle with Ménière's still active. In spite of this he runs an efficient and cheerful office, and is always planning for the Society's continued growth.

'IN FOREIGN PLACES'

by

Miss S.C.

Enfield, Middx.

I had enjoyed my lunch with some friends in the Mendana Hotel in Honiara, the capital of the Solomon Islands, where I was living and working at the time. As the four of us were leaving, strolling along the drive outside the entrance in the shade of the palm trees and bougainvillea, I began to feel increasingly unwell. I was on my way to spend the weekend with one of my lunch companions and, knowing that we had a journey ahead of us, I felt that I couldn't set out feeling so dizzy, at my friend's suggestion the two of us returned to the hotel foyer. I sat in one of the armchairs while she went and found me a drink of water. As she had some unfinished business to complete she left me there with her shopping to look after while she set off again hoping that she would return to find me feeling better.

However, things did not go according to plan and I rapidly felt worse. As I leaned back in the armchair and sat looking up at the carved roof I found that Mendana's head above me seemed to be moving round alarmingly. More urgently though I realized that I was feeling very sick so I stood up to go across the foyer to the toilets only to find that I couldn't possibly walk anywhere safely. I knew that I would fall over if I took even one step so I hastily sat down again and grabbed a plastic bag out of my luggage just in time. I sat for a while quietly vomiting into my bag while people sat around in the other chairs or wandered past giving me only a passing glance as though what I was doing was just the normal way to behave! Finally I managed to attract the attention of one of the hotel staff and when he came across to see what was wrong I hastily explained my need for another plastic bag. With considerable presence of mind he dashed into the hotel gift shop and emerged almost at once with one of their bags which I immediately started to use. Bag number one I handed to another member of staff who came up at that moment to try and sort the situation out.

Once I had managed to explain my predicament the staff could not have been more helpful. They took me back to the place where I was staying by taxi, keeping me well supplied with plastic bags all the way and literally took me and put me on the bed when we arrived. Much later in the afternoon the friend who had left me sitting in the hotel caught up with me and her shopping, though the weekend visit had to be abandoned of course. Although, I did not know it at the time I had just had my first Ménière's attack. It was also the first (and hopefully the last) time that I had been out to lunch and handed the meal back to the management in a plastic bag before leaving!

'THE SURVEYOR'S STORY'

by

Mr. E.Z.

Isle of Wight.

On the 20th February 1970 I saw an ENT specialist, as I had become aware of some hearing loss and had been sick. Almost immediately after I was in Malta and then in Hong Kong, as a land and engineering surveyor, and then travelled on to Australia. Whilst in Hong Kong I was surveying the route for a motorway around Kowloon, using Chinese engineering students to help take some profiles of steep rocky hillsides. On one occasion I had to rescue a student who had got stuck on an outcrop, but I experienced a decidedly giddy spell and was more than fortunate in being able to climb down again without falling off.

Shortly after my return to the UK in September 1970, I lost my balance and was violently sick at work and taken by ambulance to hospital. I was falling to the left although only my right ear was affected. Ménière's was thought to be the cause and was later confirmed by tests. That same month I had a grommet inserted in my right ear. Numerous attacks of giddiness followed accompanied by sickness, blurred vision, facial numbness, earache, light headedness, eye-ache, buzzing noises and neck-ache, on average several times a week. On New Years Eve 1970 at my request the grommet was removed, but the attacks still continued, some bouts of giddiness lasting for 24 hours non-stop. I also once again experienced migraine which first attacked me in the 1950's.

On the 6th August 1973 I had all my teeth removed. The decision to have this done was twofold. At the time I was also suffering from considerable tooth and jaw ache and was desperate to try anything. I had read somewhere that the fillings in one's teeth could have a very damaging effect health-wise and that their removal could be beneficial. Unfortunately the exercise had no effect in curing or even reducing my Ménière's, but at least I no longer have to experience the unsettling motion of the dentist's chair, although the rotating and tilting of a barber's chair can be upsetting.

The attacks continued on a reduced scale for the rest of the 70's and early 80's.

In January 1985 I had a bad attack and fell to the right, then in February without warning, the pattern changed dramatically with the onset of a split second drop attack - falling against the sideboard. I hardly think that 'fall' is the correct word, for it felt as though an all-in wrestler had hurled me across the room. It required an operation for a displaced cheekbone and four fractures - including the wiring up of my eyebrow. Having recovered from that I had another drop attack in May and gashed my forehead and nose on a fence post.

In that year I invested in a private hearing aid and could hear reasonably well for the first time for ages. I had previously tried Health Service aids in both ears but with not much success. I have a 90% loss in my right ear and a 70% loss in the left and cannot obtain maximum volume without experiencing feed-back and the accompanying whistling sound. TV sub-titles for me are now invaluable for the average programme is quite meaningless - rather like the old silent films but without their humour. I view the loop system with mixed blessings for TV watching, for then one cannot hope to hear what someone else in the room is saying.

I believe that the root cause of my trouble was due to the fact that during 1940 in London I found myself in the middle of a stick of five bombs, the nearest exploding just ten yards from where I was standing. No warning had been sounded and there was no opportunity to drop flat on the ground. The blast carried me through the door of a house and halfway up the staircase inside. Miraculously I was unmarked, but thought I had been decapitated, and had a very stiff neck for several weeks. Years later an X-ray revealed a wasted disc in my neck, now resulting in osteo spondilitis, and a possible cause of some of the giddiness I experience. Service during the last war as an artillery surveyor, including such battles as El Alamein and Cassino, did not do my hearing any good either.

I had two brief attacks in 1986 and 1987 - when I retired - but since then have been free of Ménière's; I do however still get signs of migraine.

On the 17th November 1989 I climbed Tryfan, a 3010 foot mountain in Snowdonia, with my grandson aged 7. There was some rock scrambling, but apart from some unsteadiness whilst "boulder hopping" I was OK. This has done a lot for my morale. I am a member of the Scottish Mountaineering Club, and during 1951 and 1952 whilst climbing on Mt. Kenya and in the Ruwenzori, I would be struck by sudden headaches and sickness - not to be confused with mountain sickness.

The term "vertigo", whilst being correct in the true medical sense, does, I think in most people's minds conjure up a "fear of heights". As a mountaineer that is certainly not true in my case, although since the onset of Ménière's I had to take extra care where I placed myself. Whilst rock climbing remained out of the question, I have done roof-top surveys (always having a secure hold nearby) and scaled ladders (with extreme caution). It is for the foregoing reason that I referred to my "bouts" as "giddiness" rather than "vertigo".

After 21 years experience of Ménière's. the most disabling effect has been the almost total hearing loss - making communication extremely difficult, and now over the telephone almost impossible. Losing one's balance into the bargain rubs salt into the wound. Music is now quite tuneless, but thankfully I can still hear the birds singing and my eyesight is sound. One just has to learn to adjust and most importantly to keep a sense of humour.

'THE WALKING STICK'

by

(Anon)

The consultant came on Monday morning at 8 o'clock. It as a week after my admission; a week of tests, uncertainty and fear. He was kind, but the blow still shocked. "The labyrinthectomy of five months ago has not been successful", he said. "There are still pockets of activity in the inner ear, causing you the same symptoms of dizziness and vomiting".

I stared at him, empty. There was nothing to say. He spoke again. "There is another way, but it means another doctor, another hospital and another operation. It involves opening the cranium and cutting the vestibular nerve to sever the connection between the diseased ear and the brain".

I wanted to scream, but nothing came out. He said, "Think about it", and, as he left, "You can go home today". I lay back on the hard hospital pillows and stared at the ceiling. Then the tears came. Hot and salty, they streamed as I sobbed uncontrollably. The nurses wanted to help, but how could they? Eventually, one came with some strong coffee and said, "You must stay one more day and the consultant will come back tomorrow to talk with you".

The rest of that day passed forlornly. I tried to read, but the dizziness forced me to stop. I talked to the nurses until lip-reading gave me a headache.

The consultant came, as promised, the next day. He tried to explain, but I was still upset. "How am I going to get home now?" I said. "How am I going to get to work? I can't walk straight, and I bump into lamp-posts!". He looked at me. "Of course", he said. "I am sorry. I will get you a walking stick".

“No, no, no!” I said, “Please not a walking stick!”. The consultant sat on my bed. “Imagine a bicycle”, he said. “Two wheels are not very stable. But add a third wheel and you find that the tricycle is much more stable than the bicycle. Imagine your walking stick as a third leg!”. He went, and I was happy again. He would arrange the new operation, and in the meantime, I had a walking stick. The physiotherapist brought the walking stick. She measured me, and chopped a bit off the end. My walking stick had to be customized. I packed my bag, and set off, walking stick in action. It saw me safely to the station by taxi and thus home by train.

Every day, I used my walking stick. It took me to the station each morning and onto the train for London. It then led me to the Red Arrow bus, where it served a most useful purpose of supplying an instant seat when the bus was full. It steadied me when the surroundings started to spin out of control, and protected me from numerous lamp-posts.

Three months later, I had the new operation - but that is another story. It was seven months before I hung up the walking stick in the coat cupboard with its redundancy note. It is still there, four years on. Will I ever throw it away? I think not. My walking stick gave me hope, courage, and the confidence to tackle what I believed to be impossible.

'THE LOSS OF MUSIC'

By

Mr. D.S.

London

In the end it did not come as a shock that I would no longer be able to listen to music. My hearing had fluctuated for a few years, but life without music, that most precious expresser of emotions, is not something I would recommend to anyone.

I was born just after the Second World War and music became my great passion from an early age. After completing my studies I became a music and English teacher in the late sixties. Monsieur Ménière did not pay his first visit to me until the early eighties and initially my hearing loss was so small as to be negligible. Then it deteriorated in my right ear and for a few years I always sat in committees, meetings, theatres and concerts, as well as when I was teaching, with the bulk of the action on my left.

Although from the beginning both of my ears had been affected, there was always the possibility that I would lose as much hearing in my left as I had in my right. It happened one night after being at the opera. - the next morning there was no more music. I now had to take up the challenge of life as a person with very little hearing. Hearing aids and other technology for the deaf have certainly made life easier. I can usually make out what people are saying although all voices have a strangely neutral distorted quality.

In August 1990 I was given a medical retirement from my job as a music teacher and knowing that I did not have the stamina to maintain any full-time work, I embarked upon a freelance approach to life. I have returned to part-time teaching, mainly of English, in an individual tuition unit where most of the difficulties imposed on my hearing by classroom teaching are conspicuously absent. I mark music examination papers at home and enjoy it because I can use my mind's ear rather than the physical one. I do a little voluntary work including some for the Ménière's Society. Lastly I try to ensure that I maintain the right balance between work, rest, and recreation. None of these now involves active music and I would never have chosen the life I now lead, but I have proved that having Ménière's disease and living a fulfilling life are not mutually exclusive.

I have a wonderful wife and enjoy travelling, walking and watching as much cricket as possible. Strangely the sounds of the bat on ball seems the same as it always did - and that is sweet music indeed.

'BEWARE THE RESETTLEMENT COURSE!'

By

Mrs. M.B.Nobbs. MBE.

Framfield, East Sussex.

George La Touche, a Guernseyman, was a tomato grower by trade when he first experienced the symptoms of the Ménière's Syndrome. Ménière's was confirmed by his local doctor after very extensive tests. He was even sent to Colchester, England, for a period where he had painful lumbar injections for testing. His hearing gradually went which was difficult to bear because there was no one in his family with the understanding and patience to help him. The only local organisation who could advise on hearing impairment was a Deaf Club and although he joined for a while he was a complete outsider. The members were all totally deafened and practised the sign language which George, of course, did not understand. He felt very alone and isolated. He wrote to The British Association of the Hard of Hearing and made many pen friends. After attending one of the Conferences and meeting all these friends he eventually married and settled in this country. For a while he struggled in his trade and coped with the Ménière's attacks as best he could. There was no Ménière's Society then to help him, his wife and friends. He wondered if the humid atmosphere of the greenhouses was aggravating his condition and thought that perhaps a change of job was necessary. He loved his creative work and reluctantly went for advice from a Disablement Resettlement Officer on the possibility of changing his line of work. An offer was accepted to go on a Resettlement Course which meant going to a residential centre a long way from home. He could only come home one weekend in three, which to him was a distressing imposition. To add to his frustrations, none of the lecturers understood his communication problem. By this time he was experiencing severe tinnitus with a profound hearing loss. He was persevering with a private hearing aid but many sounds were either very distorted or painful to hear. Consequently he suffered frequent attacks of vertigo, nausea and sickness whilst at the centre. This meant he lost out on the lectures and practical work sessions.

The Course was for about 8 weeks, by the end of which period he came home shattered, having learnt very little or having any opportunity to discuss his abilities or try any practical subjects like woodwork or painting and decorating which he liked to do.

The final assessment of him was almost negative. The Assessors said that car maintenance was not possible because of the risk of vertigo; painting and decorating had to include the ability to work on the outside of buildings and climbing ladders would be a risk employers would not want to take.

The only recommendation was a job as a STOREMAN! It was obvious no thought had gone into his communication problem. He had never progressed far with his communication skills as a good lip-reader, so how could he possibly have done well in this role? It would only have frustrated him more.

The local Disablement Resettlement Officer had the problem of finding some employment for George, who finished the last few years of his life as a cleaner in a Junior School, a big drop in status after being a skilled professional in knowing every aspect of growing, avoiding disease and practising the best ways to produce first-class tomatoes acceptable in any market in the world.

'DISASTER UNHEARD'

by

John Myall

Chobham, Surrey.

Reproduced by kind permission of "Network" the official newsletter of the National Association of Deafened People.

That particular Monday morning started off badly and got progressively worse.

I woke up feeling sick and dizzy, I was having yet another attack of Ménière's disease. To add to the fun, there is a feeling of intense pressure in the head, the tinnitus screams and what little hearing I possess drops dramatically. There was nothing my wife could do to help so she went off to work as usual and I feverishly crawled back to bed to await the uneasy sleep that when it comes brings swirling nightmares.

I eventually awoke about midday still feeling groggy but a decided improvement and headed towards the kitchen for a cup of tea. Passing the front door I stopped to retrieve a scrap of paper that had been thrust through the letter flap. With stunned horror I read its message.

THE DAMAGE TO YOUR BUNGALOW WAS CAUSED BY A LORRY REGISTRATION NUMBER ..... BELONGING TO .....

and signed by the site manager of a small building site further up the lane.

The thought of tea was forgotten and I hurriedly dressed

with sickening apprehension then sped out to see what catastrophe had befallen.

At first glance everything seemed normal, the garden wall was intact, the garage was intact - but there it was - the overhead power cable to the bungalow from a telegraph pole nearby in the lane lay draped across the garage roof. Looking at the pole from a different angle it was obviously no longer as vertical as it should be. It appeared that a heavy builder's lorry had hit the pole which stretched the cable and pulled it down.

I turned to face the bungalow but there was no sign of damage, yet something was not quite right, something was missing. The power cable had been attached to the chimney stack - "The chimney stack!!!! Where was it???? It had gone!!!!"

Rushing round to the side passageway, and there it was on the ground a heap of brick, broken tiles, twisted guttering, a demolished rainwater butt and a dangling end to the power cable that may well be very much alive.

Although most of the stack was on the ground, there was an ugly hole in the roof where the rest of it had crashed through. I dashed back into the lounge where the plaster ceiling was miraculously unscathed, but there on the carpet in front of the hearth, was soot and more rubble that had tumbled down the chimney. Next visit, the loft. Lofts are usually dark places but they become surprisingly light and airy when there is a gaping hole in the roof. The heavy loft floor boards had prevented the wreckage from battering its way into the lounge below, and that was the good news. The bad news was the view through the hole, the heavy leaden sky full of impending rain.

"What to do?" There was no chance of making a phone call, my hearing had not yet recovered sufficiently to use my amplified set, not that it really mattered, the phone line had come down as well. In times of emergency my faithful course of action is a cup of tea, a cigarette, and do some clear thinking. The electric kettle wouldn't work, no power! At least there was one piece of luck, we have a gas cooker.

The stunned brain slowly got into gear and came up with a course of action. I went to the building site and fortunately the site manager was there. He repeatedly emphasised that the accident was nothing to do with him as it had been a supplier's lorry that was involved, but - bless him - he would lend me a roofer to put a temporary patch over the hole. For the sake of simplicity I told him I had been out when it happened. Just how could I explain that I never heard the disaster or noticed the earthquake-like tremors that must have occurred.

Next came a lengthy walk down to the village store, there was no chance of getting my car out of the garage with a dodgy power cable flopping over it. I purchased a film for my camera. With an expensive accident like this, the more evidence the better, and previous experiences had taught me that there is nobody more disbelieving and unhelpful than an insurance company that thinks it may have to part with money.

Before returning to our saddened and abused home, a quick call in to a friend to ask him to phone the emergency electricity service for me. At least on getting back I was greeted by a cheery roofer who had made a start with the patch and, against all odds, the rain had held off.

My wife eventually returned home from work and listened to the incredible saga. After the photographic session I think

I deserved that next cuppa and ciggie, it is after all not every day that your house falls down around your ears and you don't know a thing about it!

'THE CROSS I HAVE TO BEAR'

by

Mrs. E.W.

Allerton, Liverpool.

War broke out when I was sixteen. At eighteen my call up papers arrived and I decided to join the Wrens. I married in 1944, my husband was serving in the RAF, and when the war ended we were demobbed. I had a medical before leaving and was pleased to be found A.1.

We were lucky enough to be granted a new council house, our son was ten months old and we were very happy. In 1950 our daughter was born and I thought "God has been good to me". My husband joined the police force, I felt very secure, then life started to change gradually.

I started having ear-aches which got so bad that the doctor sent me to the Ear, Nose and Throat clinic. A doctor there put a long thin needle into my ear, it felt as if he had pierced something, and it was so painful.

As time went on I started to have dizzy spells; I remember one day a friend called round for a chat and as I tried to get out of my chair to go and make her a cup of tea, I found I couldn't move. I felt very frightened and started to vomit, the room was whirling round. Days went by and the dizzy spells were getting worse, and all the time I was trying to look after two small children and run a home.

My balance was so affected that I could not go out alone, people thought I was drunk. If I turned my head I felt I was going to fall, so had to walk very slowly, holding on to whatever was nearby.

I was cooking the dinner one day when my husband arrived home, without thinking I turned quickly to greet him, had a dizzy spell, and went down bringing the hot frying pan with liver, onions and gravy all over my arm. My husband rushed me to the doctor, where I explained again about the dizziness, the noises and pain in my ear. He didn't examine me, just said the dizziness was due to nerves. I was convinced he was wrong and eventually he sent me to see a psychologist who did not do a bit of good.

As time went by I became depressed, I felt so sorry for my husband and children. People did not understand what I was going through, they just kept telling me to pull myself together. How could I? A clock will not work properly with the balance wheel broken. Then on top of all this, I found I was going to have another baby, - how was I going to cope? The doctor was still convinced it was nerves and said having another child might do me some good. I felt so angry!

We then had the opportunity to exchange our council house for a police house, which pleased my husband as we would be living nearer the station and it would be easier for him to keep an eye on me.

We also changed the doctor to a more local one. The new doctor thought I might be suffering from anaemia as I was bedridden at this time. The baby was due so I went into hospital and had a boy on 11th June 1959. Once again I thought how am I going to look after him? I came home, went straight to bed and the doctor treated me for anaemia, this entailed the district nurse calling round to give me liver injections. The baby hardly left my side, I would crawl to the bathroom to wash a nappy, and my mother came round as often as she could. There was a plastic sheet I would place on the bed and mother or one of the children would bring in the baby bath so I could bathe the baby myself.

I had to clothe the family by mail order and hope they would fit as shopping was out of the question. My daughter collected the groceries we needed when she arrived home from school.

My eldest son cooked the meals under my instruction after I had prepared everything. He also helped out with the washing and between the two of them they kept the house clean. I found summer the worst, as holidays were out of the question, although my husband would go back to see his family. By this time my mother had come to live with us after the death of my father, but she couldn't do much as she had a bad heart, although she was marvellous to the children, taking them on day outings.

I would watch out of the window and see the neighbours taking their children out - how I wished I could do the same!

A new doctor stopped the liver injections as they were not making any difference, but he did examine my ear which he said was perforated and thought my troubles could be Ménière's disease. I had never heard of this before and I don't think the previous doctors had either! I felt a cloud lift, maybe I will get better now. In 1960 I went to hospital for the start of many tests, hearing, ear pressure, sinuses washed out, lumber puncture etc. A top nerve specialist even confirmed my nerves were all right.

I asked "Can't you do anything for me?" The doctor said they could operate but did not like to do the operation because it would destroy the hearing in the left ear, and it was not always a success. I told him I was prepared to take the risk as I could not carry on like this any longer.

In February 1961, the night before the operation the sister asked me if I wanted a sedative. I refused and told her I was not nervous just looking forward to it. It would change our lives if it were a success ....

When I woke up in the ward after the operation, I felt as if I had been kicked in the head, but in a few days the dizziness had gone and the specialist told me to get up and walk down the ward. I was unsteady but had been told that it was to be expected. The doctors and nurses were as happy as I was.

I went home to my family, deaf in one ear. I still have noises in that ear but have learnt to live with them; the balance was not too good but I coped.

It was such a relief to get my confidence back. In 1962 I heard that they needed somebody to look after spastics for a few hours of an evening, so along with a friend, I volunteered. It proved to be a bit of a strain for my balance but I tried never to show it. We also moved house.

In 1974, my balance was getting worse, so it was back to hospital, this time seeing a different specialist for another operation. A labyrinthectomy was suggested and was not particularly successful.

In 1979, the specialist was very concerned because he knew what I had already gone through. He told me that although I did not realise it, a little bit of hearing still remained in the left ear and the only thing to be done was to sever the nerve. He said he did not like to do the operation and wanted to seek a second opinion. I asked if he had done one before, he replied "Yes two, but both were on dead bodies"! He said it was a 50/50 chance of success, but I was at the end of my tether and left the decision to him. I endured a lot more tests from the "second opinion" doctor and a date was set for the operation.

I was in hospital prepared to have the operation the following afternoon when the surgeon came to see me. He explained that it was a very delicate operation and that he would need very steady hands. He apologised that he didn't feel up to it at the time and sent me home! I was to be sent for again when the surgeon was ready.

That day finally arrived and the operation was done. I think the surgeon was relieved to find me still alive after it! He had severed the nerve leading to the brain and removed all the organs from the left ear. When I came round I noticed that my facial muscle had dropped and I couldn't close my eye!!! I looked shocking and could no longer bear to look in a mirror. When I was discharged I was on 32 tablets a day and had to wear dark glasses.

My balance still did not improve and the specialist said there was unfortunately nothing else to be done.

I tried to cope. Even simple things like ironing were difficult. I would sit on the floor, propped up against something, and do the ironing on a blanket. The small consolation was that I was eventually granted (after an appeal) Mobility Allowance.

In 1984, I suffered a heart attack and spent some time in intensive care. This was followed two years later, by the discovery that I was not making thyroid, so I am now on tablets for that for the rest of my life.

In 1985, I started to take spasm like fits, and by this time I was in a wheelchair. The ear specialist (I still continued to see him in the hope of a miracle) said it was hardening of the arteries in the neck.....He never gave me another appointment and I did not know who to turn to.....

I eventually went to see a private doctor who was convinced that my problems were coming from the ear. I have been on a wide variety of drugs, some with terrible side effects.

I still cannot sit unless I am propped up, and depend a lot on my husband (now retired) and my son. My brain is very active, I keep as cheerful as I can, and retain a sense of humour. My head never feels as if it belongs to my body and I have lost my independence. I even have to rely on my husband when I have a bath. He always used to perm my hair with a home-perm but now I have a "home-visit" hairdresser who comes when I need her. I cannot make definite appointments with her as it depends on my balance that particular day but she is good and understands my situation.

It is now 1989, I am 66 years old and have put up with this for 40 years. It seems unbelievable. My husband is 67 and I know my family have missed out on so much in life because of my illness but we have all given each other a lot of love and affection and I am proud of them. I believe that God chooses the ones to bear the cross just like Jesus.... That is my belief and it keeps me going.

Note from Terry

This was the first story I received and it so impressed on my mind the plight of the sufferer, and was the one that inspired me to make the prediction Winifred Brinson made so long ago, come true. I am glad that my promise to Mrs.E.W., of publishing her story for all to read, has at last been kept.

‘MENOPAUSE’

by

Mrs. L.T.

Huntingdon.

I am a menopausal female (physician’s designation, not mine!). This definitely adds an extra dimension to Ménière’s disease. Most mornings I rise with an unclear head, deteriorated eye-sight and not knowing whether to reach for the tablets or not. I wait until I am doing the breakfast washing up, having moved around the kitchen carefully during the breakfast preparations trying not to make any sudden turns. Hopefully, I am then struck by the first hot flush of the day, after which my head clears, the eyesight gradually improves, and I abandon any idea of taking tablets.

I cope with tinnitus by having the radio on if I am indoors, or with gardening which is such a passion, that I don’t notice it once absorbed outside. I find recruitment the worst aspect, especially the ups and downs of volume on the T and from background music. Also my husband always lowers his voice in sympathy when I have an attack and this actually makes things worse.

As for getting off to sleep at night, I read until my eyes close, but if I sit down after lunch, I have no problem nodding off. Cat-naps are best and safest using a special pillow, as I think there is a danger of my head dropping to the side when in a chair and causing neck problems.

Since moving to a quiet village in the country and giving up my stressful job as a school dinner lady, the children leaving home (although they still know where to come with their problems!), and learning how to control the attacks with medication, life is not too bad.

'FAITH IN THE FACE OF ADVERSITY'

by

Mrs. C.F.

Manchester.

I will try to tell you what happened to me the best way I can. Eight years ago when I was thirty, I started to get a constant ringing noise in my ears and head. I was also getting bad vertigo, being violently sick, falling over a lot and couldn't seem to hear properly.

After many visits to my doctor I was sent to hospital for tests and a brain scan. They eventually diagnosed Ménière's disease and prescribed tablets, but unfortunately my attacks just kept getting worse. They got so bad that I had to give up work and driving. At one time I was on fifteen tablets a day and told to rest, but with three children I found this very hard to do although I really did try as things were getting so bad.

I was sent to see a neurosurgeon in January 1989 to see if there was anything he could do. He said the only remaining option was surgery and that I might lose my hearing but at least I would be a lot better. As both ears were affected it was a big decision to take, but really there wasn't much choice as I had a young family and was fast becoming trapped indoors.

I have a very deep faith and a good and loving husband so I prayed for guidance. After a lot of discussion and soul-searching we decided it would be best to have the surgery.

I went into hospital in February 1989 where they operated on my right ear. Ten days after the operation things were still as bad. I had retained some hearing so they asked me if I would be prepared to have the left operated on. I couldn't stay like I was, so I agreed. On this occasion I lost all the hearing in the ear, but I didn't mind as it seemed a small price to pay if I was going to become better again.

You can imagine the shock I got after spending five and a half weeks in hospital, two major operations, a shaved head, a lot of pain and discomfort only to find that getting out of bed and trying to walk was impossible. I couldn't even stand by myself. When we questioned the doctors they said it would just take time.

On the day I was discharged my husband had to wheelchair me out. I felt shell-shocked to say the least, after all I had walked into hospital unaided and could not understand what was happening to me now. When we got home it took my husband and eldest daughter, who was fourteen at the time, to get me indoors. Over the following months they had to teach me to walk with the aid of two sticks, help me dress, wash, shower, and do all the housework between them.

It is nearly two years now since I had my operations and I am sorry to say that things are a lot worse than they were before. I have no sense of balance and the most I can walk is about 200 yards and that is with two walking sticks. After such a short distance I simply don't know where I am as everything is moving about. It seems as though the floor, walls, paths are jumping up and hitting me then they fly away again. It can be just as bad when I go out in a car with my husband or friends, and sometimes it even happens in my wheelchair.

The ringing noises are getting unbearable and of course the dizziness never completely leaves me. I have only a little hearing left in my right ear and we are all trying to learn sign language so we will still be able to communicate if it gets any worse. Although I take tablets to try and control it the vomiting gets very bad and I am losing so much weight. Frequently I have to spend several days at a time in bed, and often I don't know where I am or what I am doing as my head feels as if it is on another planet. I also get violent headaches and a terrific pain behind the ears. At times I get blurred vision and if I try to focus my eyes onto something moving they go into spasms and roll round and round which makes the vertigo even worse.

I have been discharged from hospital because they tell me there is nothing more they can do and that I must come to terms with it.

I have been strongly advised not to try and go out on my own and to stay away from the cooker. There are so many other ordinary things I can't do in spite of having the house adapted where possible to make life easier. I have had handrails fitted from the front gate to the front door, a stair lift, a handrail at the top of the stairs to get off the stair life, a handrail along to my bedroom, a commode in my bedroom, and a shower cabinet fitted in my bedroom with a seat inside for me to sit on while I shower. There are also handrails from the back door to the back toilet, with a frame fixed over the toilet for me to hold on to, to help me get on and off. There is a loop system for the television, and the doorbell and telephone are adapted so that when they ring all the main lights in the house come on. The telephone is amplified. Most of these things we had to pay for ourselves as the Social Services had run out of money.

I still think I am lucky because there are a lot of people in this world who are worse off than me. I have some very good friends who help when help is needed, a loving and supportive husband and three lovely children. Even though they can't really understand what is happening to Mum they are wonderfully caring.

I have a very deep faith which helps me through the bad times, and I know that my faith will continue to give me the strength to face each new day. Along with the help of my family and friends I will continue to overcome my problem. In spite of everything I do not suffer from depressions and I will never give up hope that one day things might start to settle down and be better for myself and my family.

I pass a lot of my time by reading or knitting or going to church. I teach the young people at our church on Friday nights and once a week go to college to learn sign language.

Although the operations did not turn out the way I hoped they would, I don't feel any anger or bitterness, or any blame towards anyone and still manage to enjoy myself.

'A YOUNG MUM WITH M.D.'

by

Mrs. K.W.

Bude, Cornwall.

I am now 29 and expecting my second baby, my little boy Nathan is three. At the end of my first pregnancy I had a lot of severe tinnitus which I won't get again this time. I assume it was due to pressure towards the end of carrying the baby.

Over the 16 years I have had M.D. my symptoms have altered in some ways. The dizziness fluctuates, - it's so good to feel well for a time, then suddenly the problems are back again, and I do find that I get very "down" even though I know that this is the way it goes.

Stress and tiredness certainly don't help although they are not always easy to avoid with a family to look after. I stopped taking medication a long time ago as I felt it wasn't making any difference.

I have always worked since leaving school, full time for eight years then part time since having Nathan. There were occasions when I felt like giving it up when the M.D. was really giving me a rough time, and as a result had more than my share of time off for sickness, but I kept working as I thought that it had to be better in the long run.

I've learned to live with it the best I can, all that matters are my children being healthy. Certainly having Nathan made a significant difference in my life as I know my next one will too.

I'm sure all Mum's (and Dads) who have M.D. will know what I mean, having something really important to think about helps a lot.

* * *

'THE NIGHT OF THE SLIDE SHOW'

by

'MENDY'

"Tell me when you want the lights doused." The club secretary's question brought me back to my present task, and I looked around at a surprisingly full audience even some professional photographers of long standing; they would probably pull me to bits after the show!

The thought of this forthcoming screening had helped me the last few weeks to overcome the awful feeling of awakening each morning and trying to get to grips with normal living. Sometimes when I got to work and the day progressed the nausea would ease off and I finished up in the best of spirits, other times it got the best of me and I had to be brought home by car.

I had long been interested in photography and it was my wife who first suggested I join a camera club. I had messed around with cameras for years, my speciality being audio-visual, that is to put the sound automatically with the slides. After several years I perfected a system that was reliable and could go out and take photographs, then spend the next few weeks writing up commentaries, dubbing sound effects and adding music. I thought they were only good enough to show my immediate circle of friends but my wife was convinced they deserved a wider audience.

She had a lot to put up with these last five years since my world suddenly took a tumble. I had been feeling ill for some weeks and thinking I had flu took a few days off work. This particular day whilst on my own I suddenly felt much worse, my palms began to sweat and I was cold and uncomfortable. Suddenly the world as I knew it went haywire, silently the floor and ceiling became a jumbled mass, I fell down, arms spread out and hands grasping the carpet which was slimy with vomit; I closed my eyes to try and blot out the chaos they saw.

I crawled to the front door to get help from a passer-by or neighbour, every slight movement bringing on a fresh wave of nausea. How long it took to get the door open I can't remember, but I finally made it and slid out on to the cold concrete step. At last I attracted the attention of a neighbour and was relieved that I would soon get medical help. Then came the total disbelief, laying on the doorstep, hearing the neighbour on the phone being told by the doctor's surgery that they didn't want to know, and to phone for an ambulance.

I woke up in hospital the next day feeling no after effects, and being told I had Ménière's disease. It was six months later that I got my next attack and as time went by they got more frequent. M.D. became printed on my everyday living.

I nodded to the secretary and the lights dimmed, the intro music swelled up and the title glowed on the screen - "Traction Engine Rally", nothing complicated, no special sound effects just music and commentary. A murmur of appreciation went through the audience at the end, followed by hoots of derision when I announced the next would be my holiday in East Anglia. They all knew the ones of little Johnny on the beach digging sand castles with Mum.

The holiday slides showed a trip round Happisburgh, Overstrand, Norwich Cathedral and its surroundings, plus some of the local pubs, with a short story interspersing the music. Then came a fresh tape and a new magazine of slides for the projector "How I clicked in Spain", the music giving the mood of the country then breaking to the cries of "Ole" from the crowd at the bull-fight.

I was feeling proud and pleased with myself as I started on the last magazine "London Docks". The enthusiastic reception from the audience completely drove from my mind the nagging terror of impending attacks that were becoming all too frequent now. I had worked since I was fourteen, working my up from the shop floor to manager then, unable to carry on because of the Ménière's, I was forced to resign and take a job as a handyman.

The last magazine and tape came to an end, the lights went on and the secretary came over to thank me. He said this was a new dimension for the club which to date had always specialised in developing, printing and the occasional silent slide show. My effort in mixing the commentaries, sound effects and music were thoroughly enjoyed.

As we drove home I was on a high, emotion welled up and I glanced at my wife who had put up with so much these last few years, cancelled holidays, weddings, parties, yet she never complained. "Could I have put up with so much if it had been her?" I felt very ashamed, but I doubted it, as much as I loved her.

In the excitement of the evening I had forgotten about that "shushing" noise in my right ear, and everything associated with it, surely the bad times were over and the future was looking good.

A couple of weeks later as I got ready for work, I was feeling a little unsteady but this was nothing unusual, I realised my ears were making a lot more noise and that sound seemed to be closing down. At work I found myself with sweating palms again and the head feeling floppy, - signs I knew too well. I spoke to my workmates but could not understand their replies. and their expressions indicated that I was shouting; the noise in my head confused all sounds, then came the vertigo and the panic, - once again the future was not looking quite so good. Two of my workmates drove me home then half carried and half dragged me up the path, into the house and laid me on the sofa. Fortunately my wife was there and fetched blankets as I was shivering badly and as usual took on that horrible deathly pallor, but at least she knew I was best left alone. It subsided enough for me to get to bed after a couple of hours and there I had to stay for three weeks!

When I felt able to get up the brass band that had been playing in the middle of my head had disappeared, and the rushing and throbbing noises in the ears was at a lower level but all sound was now a mish-mash of discord. Even trying to read was an effort.

Gingerly as I walked from the bedroom I had to pass the room where I kept my photographic gear. Opening the door I looked at the projector as it stood on the bench. Alongside was the recording equipment cold and silent. The sounds of cars, ships, street scenes and music were for me now an unintelligible noise. The night of the slide show had been one of my great achievements and at the same time a swan song.

Emotion welled up then the nausea came again, all I was fit now was to totter towards the toilet and vomit!.

'THERE IS LIFE AFTER MENIERE'S DISEASE'

by

Mrs. Barbara Parkinson.

Poynton, Cheshire.

Twelve years ago I was diagnosed as having Ménière's disease. Having worked in the medical profession for many years I did have an inkling of what it was but had no idea how much it was going to affect the rest of my life. I was in my early 30's at the time with two energetic toddlers and a part time job as a radiographer in a busy Casualty department and as you can imagine life became very difficult.

I will not bore you with my symptoms and subsequent treatment, I'm sure many of you could recount pretty much the same story. Eventually I had a Nerve Section on my left ear. Six months later I couldn't believe that I was on the top of a mountain in Austria with a pair of skis on my feet, this was really progress. However I was soon brought down to earth (literally). I couldn't believe my bad luck as I had started having attacks again. Ménière's disease was again diagnosed, this time in my right ear. It was very aggressive and after two unsuccessful saccus operations I was lucky if I managed to get out of bed on more than three days a week. After a lot of thought and talking with my very supportive husband and specialist I underwent a labyrinthectomy on my right ear in December 1989. I really felt that I couldn't be any worse off.

So after the initial period of readjustment after the operation, here I am with no functioning balance organs and little hearing but how wonderful, the sure knowledge that I can never have another attack. What joy to know that if I arrange to go out for lunch a week on Tuesday that I'll be able to go. OK, so I'll never be able to ski again, so much more relaxing to sit and enjoy the view and watch the world go past with a good book in one hand a glass of wine in the other. I'll never be able to play badminton or listen to music or go to the theatre again. I have now become quite creative and spend many happy hours doing tapestries. I'm also about to embark on a new career, doing a correspondence course in chiropody. Now that I'm no longer able to drive, as I have to be stationary to focus, I've discovered the pleasure of walking which is just as well, because for the past two years I've been the proud owner of a Hearing Dog for the Deaf. What a difference Wockie has made to my life. My confidence when I was alone in the house had gone completely. I missed telephone calls and often the first I would know about a caller was a face at the window. All that is now a thing of the past. Wockie alerts me to all the sounds I no longer hear, the ringing telephone, a knock at the door, the alarm clock and the smoke detector. He has also got me out into the outside world again as I am now in great demand as a speaker to various groups, schools etc. We are welcomed wherever we go. Talk about every cloud has a silver lining! It couldn't be truer in my case. We enjoy some lovely walks and in a way being deaf brings to your notice again all the things that you haven't perhaps noticed for a while and you learn to take pleasure from things not related to sound.

I suppose the turning point for me in accepting what had happened to me was joining a lip-reading class. I would encourage anyone with a hearing loss however slight to go along. Don't do as I did and wait until it is a necessity. It is your insurance policy for the future. I made a lot of new friends and what a relief to meet people with similar problems. There was even a Ménière's sufferer in the class the first I'd met! What a lot of fun we had while learning a new skill which can make all the difference to everyday life. I'm now quite a competent lip-reader but still make terrible gaffes like the unforgettable day when I mistook “wines of a certain age are vintage” for “wives of a certain age are frigid”!

So yes, there is life after Ménière’s disease. It’s certainly different, but with the love and support of family and friends I am now thoroughly enjoying life. I’ve always been a firm believer that life is what you make it. It’s no good wishing for what might have been. So take heart, always think that tomorrow will be better and it probably will be.

'COPING'

by

Mrs. E.G.

Roscrea, Eire.

I am 65 and have had Ménière's for 28 years. An eminent specialist in Dublin assured me I would never die from it, but he neglected to say that it would cause havoc and devastation to my life.

I attended him for quite a while in between bouts of remission. He tried me on various tablets, but the attacks increased and I was eventually in bed more than being up and around. So I had the destruction operation on the affected ear, severing the nerve. It of course made that ear deaf and affected my eyes. I had to wear dark glasses to help.

Things did improve but then came the menopause and this didn't help.

As time went on I tried various medications but ended up with Stugeron, and Mogadon at night. Unbelievably I had claustrophobia and agoraphobia at the same time, coupled with disorientation and agitation. I'm sure I would have gone mad had it not been for my devoted husband.

I no longer drive, so after my husband died twelve years ago, it became imperative to sell my home and move to an apartment with everything nearby, post office, doctor, grocer, chemist, newsagent etc. I have a large grown family and now live quietly. I make myself go out regularly and try to go a little further each time, but I don't go out of town as I need to have the street walls handy if only to give me confidence.

'DANCE MACABRE WITH MR. MENIERE'

by

Ms.S.C.

Warsaw, Poland.

Thirty years ago I was a young girl, my hearing wasn't good but not so bad, but deafness was beginning. One day in May 1960 I went camping with some friends. All of a sudden I felt strange and had difficulty in turning my head, the earth and all the trees in the forest were beginning to dance with me. This dance Macabre lasted for two days and I hadn't any idea what was wrong with me. My friend joked "Sabina is drunk".

Some years passed and my hearing grew progressively worse. Between 1960 and 1970 this dance Macabre recurred several times. I live in Warsaw and sought medical help. Hungarian Stugeron and Polish Aviomarin tablets were prescribed, but for a bad attack I was given Fenactil which made me so sleepy, and made it so difficult to think, that I could not function normally and was obliged to reduce my work to four or five hours a day.

My financial situation became bad, I spent a long time immobilised in bed.

"There are no efficacious medicines for Ménière's disease" said the doctors. "It is the result of your growing deafness, you must rearrange your life-style, avoid bending and don't move your head more than necessary".

I was shocked, particularly as I lived alone and had no-one to help me.

At about this time I heard about a neighbour who had been

suffering from vertigo for ten years, she was operated on for cancer in her head........ I was 45 years old and so much wanted to live ...... and live normally.

The worst arrived one night in 1986. In the evening all was OK. and I read before going to sleep, and feeling perfectly well. At about two o' clock I awoke with my head feeling hot, and my room began to dance with me. There was a bad feeling in my throat and I vomited once, twice, three times ...... "It is the end, please God don't leave me I pray to you". I couldn't get out of bed, or even turn my head a centimetre to the left or right, I was powerless. I wept. This state lasted for about 30 hours. After a long sleep in an uncomfortable position I found with great relief that at last I was able to wash myself. I then sat in my armchair and thought; "Dear God, you have given me a chance to live, I thank you". I made an effort to watch the TV. but it was impossible my eyes would not focus. I slept all next day, I was so tired, as if having made a great physical effort.

After three days I decided to go to a neighbour. "Help me please, I suffer from Ménière's disease, telephone the doctor". She did this and the doctor came looked into my eyes examined my deafness invalidity papers and said, "Madam, you suffer from vertigo and must learn to live with it. I will give you a certificate for six days off work and a prescription for Fenactil, Stugeron and Aviomarin!!

After five days it was a little better so I went back to work. Often I had the impression that my chair would slide with me, it was a nasty feeling. I didn't talk about my illness in the office as I had no wish to be called a hysterical women, which is often the case with these symptoms. Those who do not suffer from loss of balance have no real understanding of its meaning. As we say, "People who don't eat oranges don't know the flavour".

The great attack of 1986 has not repeated itself, but I have many "little problems" with my balance, but worse than that is my profound deafness.

* * *

'THE PLUMBER'S STORY'

by

Mr. M.B.

Watford, Herts.

When I was a plumber in 1973 I was working on a back boiler in a house, when all of a sudden the room went upside down and I was sick all over the lady's carpet. I remember her asking my mate "Has he been drinking"?

I just couldn't stop being sick and eventually my mate brought me back home, put me to bed, and my wife called the doctor. He diagnosed Ménière's disease.

I got over this attack and presumed that that was that, and thought no more about it, - until six months later the same thing happened again. There had been a buzzing in my right ear for some time, but now it was getting so loud that I had trouble hearing with it, not that it mattered too much because the left ear was good.

As time went by the attacks got much worse. I was sent to see a consultant, given all the various pills which didn't help, eventually going to hospital for more tests. The specialist was reluctant to operate as some hearing still remained in the affected ear.

About 18 months ago I woke up one morning with a loud

noise in my left ear this time, so I immediately went back to the hospital where it was confirmed that I now had it in both ears. The hearing has declined rapidly and at times I am almost completely deaf.

Two months ago I was driving the works van and had a very bad attack. I just managed to get home and went to bed. I haven't worked since as I feel giddy all the time. Different pills have been prescribed but with no success. I hope they will operate on my left ear which has no hearing at all, it may give me some relief.

'THE HELL OF MENIERE'S'

by

Mrs J.M.

It is now over four years since my left ear started to give me trouble. Life was running smoothly and my family were growing up, and I had found myself a job as a part time shop assistant. It was good to be amongst company and I enjoyed my work.

I did not take much notice at first when the buzzing noises started in my ear, I shrugged it off hoping it would pass over like all the other little aches and pains that come and go. Then I began to notice that the buzzing was becoming quite regular and getting louder. I even asked one of my family to put their ear close to mine and listen for the loud noise that was now with me constantly. Of course they couldn't hear anything and couldn't understand what I was talking about. Sleep was difficult and even during the day I got no relief, and soon my work began to suffer, I couldn't hold a proper conversation and concentrating was difficult.

I eventually went to the doctor and explained what was going on. She examined my ear, looking down it with a light, said she could not see anything wrong and it would probably go away. I wish it could have been that simple!

The noise would alter from time to time, changing to a high pitched screech followed by a long whining sound. I thought at one point that if it kept up I would go mental. My husband said that I must go to an ear specialist, he was getting no sleep from my constant tossing and turning, trying to get my head into a position that might quieten the constant noise in my ear. My family tried to make jokes about it, I know they were trying to take my mind off it. They would say things like “It could be the Martians trying to get in touch, you’re picking up signals from a flying saucer,” or “Mother has a built in radio in her ear, she’s trying to get “Top of the Pops”. They tried to make me laugh as I was looking so drawn and vacant.

Having decided to see a specialist I felt relieved, thinking I may get something done at last. What a waste of time and money! (I went privately). He examined my ear then said “Go to your own doctor and have your ears syringed, this will stop the noise, there’s a bit of wax there.” He mumbled this from behind his desk and I could hardly hear what he said. When I asked him to repeat it he said “Are you deaf?” I felt so embarrassed and left feeling sadder than ever. I wondered why did he not understand that I could not concentrate properly on what he was saying because the noise in my head was so loud.

I went back to work thinking I would have my ears syringed and everything would be all right, and I would be able to enjoy my work again and laugh and joke with the other women.

I made my appointment with the doctor, telling him what the specialist said. After the syringing I felt a bit dizzy but the nurse said it was quite normal and not to worry. I thought to myself that the problem may be eased at last.

The nightmare started two days later when I was at work behind the counter serving a customer. Without warning, everything went black, and for a second my brain seemed to switch off. I sank to my knees, I didn’t faint, then sat there and called out “I can’t move”. The funny thing was that in those few moments I noticed my ear had stopped buzzing. The manager came and helped me on to a chair. He tried to give me a drink but I couldn’t take it as my head was all muddled up and the eyes would not focus properly. He took me home and my husband came in shortly afterwards and sent for the doctor. At first my family thought I was having a heart attack as my chest was thumping so hard. The doctor said no, the heart was very strong but blood pressure and pulse were very high. I was told to go to bed for a few days and take tablets for blood pressure.

When I felt better I wrote to my work manager telling him that I must have been overdoing things, and that I had better give up my job. He was very understanding and said that I could come back when I felt better.

I never did go back as things went from bad to worse. As soon as my head cleared my ear would start buzzing again. Then the attacks became worse and more frequent, and I was afraid to leave the house. I could be sitting having a conversation, or standing up cooking a meal when, without warning the world would start to spin. I would just whirl round in total darkness and be soaked in perspiration. This could go on for hours then I would go very cold and start to vomit. I would keep vomiting until I had nothing left inside me, and afterwards would fall into an exhausted sleep. After an attack I would feel very weak and my head would seem cloudy for at least three days.

No sooner would I begin to feel right again when I would have another attack. Several times the doctor was called out but all he would say was "Just keep taking the tablets!" Never a word of what was wrong with me. I was losing weight and rapidly starting to look terrible. My family were very worried and would sit for several hours at a time nursing me through these attacks as I was so afraid when they were happening.

I think the most awful part was the spinning in total darkness, there was no way to stop it and it just seemed to go on for ever, then the heavy vomiting which I could not control. My family would have to change my clothes and clean me up so many times it must have been a nightmare for them as it was for me.

One Sunday I was just sitting when my head just fell forward and I banged it on the table. My husband managed to get me onto the sofa and sent for the doctor again, but it was such a fierce attack that I was totally unaware of what was going on.

Being a Sunday was a blessing, it was a different doctor on duty. He examined me and after hearing the symptoms told the family I had Ménière's disease. We had never heard of this before and he patiently explained everything about it. What a kind man he was. He said that the pills I was taking were of no use for Ménière's and that he would write a note to my own doctor asking him to prescribe different ones, but they would not cure me only calm things down, and the attacks would become less frequent. He then gave me an injection which was a strong dose of the tablets, and said that as I was in such a bad way it would relieve the symptoms quicker.

When the doctor had finished with me, the family could not thank him enough. For months we had all been sick with worry just not knowing what was wrong with me, fearing and imagining all kinds of dreadful things. The torment and despair that went through me because of not knowing, was awful.

I often wonder if other people have felt the same as I did at that time. Although not very pleasant, finding out exactly what was wrong at least settled the mind.

The months dragged on, I took the tablets regularly, and although the attacks still occurred, they were less frequent. I started to eat better and manage my everyday affairs easier than I had been doing before. In the past I sometimes wondered if I would simply die during an attack, unable to pull myself out of the swirling darkness. Knowing this would not happen eased my mind and took away a lot of the burden.

When I had a fierce attack, the doctor would come and give me the injection which certainly helped me to get over it. I did not dare stray from home, and my family worried even if I went down to the local shops by myself.

After I decided to see a specialist, I insisted the doctor refer me to a different one than I had seen before, remembering how unkind he had been.

This time it was a lady specialist, and I visited her several times to have my ears syringed and tested. She confirmed that I had Ménière's syndrome, said the attacks would diminish, I would go completely deaf and that there was nothing that could be done about it; I would just have to cheer up and learn to live with it.

After that I thought "You are now on your own, it will be up to you to sort yourself out".

Sitting alone one day in my bedroom, having just got over a mild attack - a "decent" one I used to call them then if I didn't go completely out - I came to a decision. I must fight this thing or just give in to it and become a recluse, afraid to wander very far, and no holidays because of the fear of having an attack among strangers. No, I was going to fight and try to live some sort of normal life, in preference to what I was living then.

I thought it all out in my mind, first I would start to go out more, a little further each day, then I would try the town centre. The first time I went to the town, my daughter Pauline insisted on going with me as it was a bus ride away. On reaching the town, the noise and the traffic really got to me, and it took quite a while to adjust myself, - a problem I still have even now. All went well for a while then I fell down, banging my head on the pavement, wrenching my shoulder and bruising my knees. My daughter sat beside me and cried. An ambulance took me to hospital and I spent the next four days there having X-rays and check-ups. I was lucky that nothing was broken, but after this first visit to town since the attacks first started, I arrived home in a taxi with a lump on my forehead, my left arm in a sling and my knees bandaged up.

My family were speechless as I walked in, but before any of them could utter a word I said, "Don't say anything. I refuse to listen to you telling me not to go to town again, I'm determined to beat this thing and I'm not giving up". Of course they were worried for me, but they admired my courage.

As soon as I was fit again, back to the town I went. Pauline escorted me again and this time there were no complications.

I did not want to have an operation on the ear, but thought to myself, "Why not try some old-fashioned remedies?" After all, how did people manage in olden times? Surely Ménière's existed then although they may not have understood what it was. I went to the library and second hand book shops searching for old fashioned remedy books, and came home with quite a good selection. My family were delighted and relieved with my safe arrival home, this being only my second time into town alone.

What I did discover on my outings was that strong sunlight and the fluorescent lighting in big stores bothered me. My head became muddled and I found it difficult to concentrate.

On my next visit to the doctor I mentioned this to him. He was very understanding, and suggested that I wear sun glasses to see if this would help. I had a bit of a problem trying to find any that would suit as the ordinary sunglasses seemed to be of no use. On mentioning this to a neighbour, she said she had a very dark pair that had belonged to her late husband, and did I want to try them? They were perfect and I wore them often.

At first my family thought this was hilarious, they started singing Roy Orbison's songs and asked me if I wanted a guitar. They were always trying to joke to cheer me up, and now when I look back I realise what a marvellous family I had.

What fun we had trying the old fashioned remedies! I read one book that suggested that noises in the ear meant insanity, what a shocker that was! I ignored that one and tried the next. I was amazed at the "cures" of olden-times and tried herbs of all descriptions. Sometimes one of the family would pop into my bedroom to check on me during the night, after having tried out another queer recipe during the day, they would worry in case it had any side effects. I tried to explain that all these herbs were harmless and I would certainly not have used them otherwise. I did have cause for doubt on one remedy that needed hemp seed. Getting quite brave with my town excursions, I went to a large chemist and asked for hemp seed. The assistant went to ask the pharmacist then the next I saw was him flouncing out from the back of the shop. He looked me up and down and said angrily that they did not sell that sort of thing. I fled from the shop feeling very embarrassed but when I told my family about the incident they went into hysterics. We all wondered if it was some sort of drug and the pharmacist thought I was going to smoke it. Needless to say I never tried asking for it again.

One of the remedies I kept to myself and tried out in secret, afraid that the family would begin to suspect my sanity. One said that your own spittle used every morning as soon as you woke up had been known to cure all kinds of maladies. I tried this for weeks, wetting my finger in my mouth and rubbing it round my ear; had another attack so threw that one out. My ear still buzzed but I was learning to ignore it.

Another book suggested that we are ruled by the moon, and in order to rid ourselves of maladies, every time there is a full moon one must bow to it three times and ask it to take away the affliction. I had to sneak out into some quiet corner of the garden at night to try this one out, but try it I did. For three full moons this went on but my ear still buzzed and I felt such a fool.

It was during this time that my daughter Lorna told me that she was going away for a few weeks holiday, touring in France. She returned with a joyful smile on her face, the main purpose of her trip had been to go to Lourdes and bring some Holy Water back for me to try. It was a large canister and she said "with your great faith and belief mother I know this will cure you". All the family gathered around as she poured me a full glass. The looks on their faces as I drank could not possibly be described, I am sure they were all expecting a bolt of lightning to shoot across the sky.

I had always had a sincere belief in the miracles of Lourdes and my daughter told me about her visit there, people who were terribly ill and maimed queuing up for hours to be bathed in the water. Some spent all night waiting to be blessed by the priest. As I listened to her story I thought of these people and then of myself. "How could I, with only Ménière's syndrome ask to be cured when there were so many others with far worse ailments?" God must surely see to them first, I felt very humble, and because I loved my daughter dearly I could not tell her my thoughts. I promised I would drink the water regularly and I did.

I still kept trying my secret remedies, my ear still buzzed, but the really bad attacks were becoming more spaced out. I could go out much more and my youngest daughter Sharron had taken to going on long walks with me in the evenings after she finished work. This was something she dared not do previously, being afraid that I would fall down.

I was beginning to feel much better in myself, so much so that I thought "Why not try a holiday?" I talked it over with my husband and family and they all thought it was a good idea and felt sure it would do me good. We saw a holiday advertised in the local paper for a coach tour in Italy, it seemed to be just the thing as we all loved bus excursions.

It was to be a foursome Lorna, Sharron, my husband and myself. When we set off we were all very excited and the first part of the journey was lovely. We crossed the Channel on the boat with no problems, - then came the Alps - What a disaster!

I never gave it a thought that we would have to go through the Alps to get to Italy, but even if I thought about it I would still not have realised that the altitude might affect me, I was too excited about going. When we got to the Alps, the driver stopped the bus for us to get out to view the glaciers on the mountains. I thought it was a lovely idea and got out with everyone else. It was beautiful, the mountain scenery absolutely marvellous. I looked up to the mountain peaks and the next thing I knew I was staggering to the side of the bus for support, my balance had gone completely. My husband had to lift me back on board where I had one of the fiercest attacks I have ever experienced.

The family were beside themselves with worry. I looked so ghastly that the two men in charge wanted to take me to a hospital immediately. The girls refused, saying they knew what was wrong with me, but found it hard to explain. They were afraid that if I were taken to hospital I would be left there. The other passengers and drivers were marvellous! A back seat was cleared for me, everybody moved up to make this possible. They turned the music off and drove slowly and gently. I lay like this for several hours until we reached our hotel. I shall never forget those people, complete strangers who went out of their way to do things for me.

I was carried straight up to my hotel room leaving the others to sort out the booking and luggage. After a sleep I was much better, but weak and if I had been at home would have stayed in bed, but being on holiday I made myself get up next morning. Everyone was surprised to see me when I went into the dining room. I felt dreadful, but could not spoil the holiday for the rest, so tried my best to hide it.

I sat alone on the beach for most of the time although I still felt ill. I had another attack later on in the week, and the family were frantic with worry about how I would manage the homeward journey. I got up again and tried to act as normal as possible, doing a little shopping and some sightseeing with my husband. I told the girls to go off and enjoy themselves, and that I would be all right with their father staying with me. I felt sad more than anything else as I knew that it was spoiling their holiday.

Then came the time for the journey home. I was still feeling weak and ill but pretended to be all right and able to travel. When we reached the mountains, one of the passengers suggested I plug my ears with cotton-wool and put a coat over my head. We thought that if I had my ears blocked up for the pressure change, and couldn't see the mountains it might help. Strangely enough it worked as I didn't have an attack, not even a mild one.

Although my body still felt a total shambles, after the Alps, I was able to sit quietly and watch the passing scenery, and on the Channel ferry, even managed a light meal. I slept most of the time on the last lap.

On arriving at our local bus station, my son Raymond was there to meet us and take us home in his car. He looked at me and said "Good grief, mother, how ill you look". I replied, "Just get me home Ray and I'll be fine in no time at all". The girls explained what had happened, and he made me promise not to go to any mountainous regions again. I said I was still not going to give in to Ménière's, but would keep to flat lands in future.

It took two or three weeks to get back to my normal self. My daughters said they loved Italy but would never do anything like that again.

During this period of recovery, Lorna sat with me to have a chat. She said, "Mother, when I bought the Holy Water back from Lourdes I was so happy, I was convinced that this was the answer. Now when I look back at you, knowing your belief in God, I feel sad. I am beginning to wonder about my faith, if God listens to everybody why hasn't he listened to you?" I was shocked that she should feel this way and not sure what to say, but knew that I had to give her some explanation. I told her of the suffering and heartaches of other people and this made me feel unjustified in asking for a cure as there were so many others in need. She was stunned with disbelief, saying she had gone to Lourdes, and now I could not find it in myself to ask God for a cure.

I then realised just how upset she was, and how thoughtless I must have seemed to her. There and then I made my decision, I went upstairs to my bedroom, took the Holy Water in my hands, went down on my knees and prayed to God for a cure from Ménière's.

It is now over a year since I had a bad attack. My ear still buzzes from time to time but only on the days when I am feeling a bit run down. The rest of the time it is quite normal and I can go out and about whenever I want to. Strong sunlight still bothers me, but I have my dark glasses to get around this problem, which is really quite small when I think how bad things were in the past.

I can now do so many things that were impossible before. For instance, I could not stand near water, lakes, swimming pools or any kind of water that flowed or rippled. This movement always affected my balance. I could only look at water from a distance. Now, I regularly go to our local pool and have learnt to swim quite well, what is more I really enjoy it.

My family are now settling in to their own lives. Lorna has moved into her own house, something she has waited a long time for but kept putting it off because she didn't want to leave me. Ray went to London and got a good job there. Sharron, my youngest, who had been longing for some time to live and work in France, went there with a light heart because she saw me looking my old self again. I have actually travelled to France twice on my own to visit her. It is lovely to go visiting friends and relatives with my husband and not have them running round to me because I am not well again.

It is just my husband and myself at home now and we are happy to live a normal life. I thank God that I have had a wonderful family, because without them I am certain I would have given in and gone completely downhill.

Every day I still dab a little Holy Water in my ear and thank God for listening to me - I know he did.

This story is dedicated to my family who suffered with me, especially my daughters, Lorna and Sharron, who insisted I write this story in the hope that it may in some way help other Ménière's sufferers.

'BURNT OUT MENIERE'S'

1943 - 1989

by

Mrs. P.G.

Fakenham, Norfolk.

In 1943, the first indication I had of any symptom was a pronounced ringing/whistle in the right ear. I consulted my GP. who syringed the ear, but the noises continued.

Two years later I started to have frequent attacks of giddiness with nausea and vomiting. These were diagnosed as "stomach upsets" and I was prescribed flatulence medicine for about a year.

In 1946 I moved from Basingstoke to Eastleigh, and my new GP. sent me to the ENT department at a nearby hospital. There I had my nostrils cauterised and a minor operation to remove a piece of bone from one of them. The attacks continued to occur at approximately weekly intervals, but not to any set pattern.

In 1947 I moved to Surrey and my new GP. diagnosed Ménière's disease, and referred me to the local ENT department. There I was seen by a consultant who began to treat me at his clinic at a hospital in London.

I was given a full range of tests, nicotinic acid tablets and tranquillising pills, but not much information. Eventually my attacks became less and less frequent and I decided to start a family. During my pregnancy they petered out entirely and, a few months after the birth of my baby, I was discharged from the outpatients clinic, but still with a continuous whistle in my right ear. No information about possible deafness was given, probably not much was known then.

From 1950 I lead a normal life, brought up three children and later worked as a nursery nurse, becoming matron, until I retired in 1988. Sometime during those years it became evident that I was losing hearing in my right ear. After tests, I was told that nothing could be done and I now have practically no response at all in that ear.

However, in 1970 my job became very stressful and I started having dizzy spells again. When they became quite frequent I was referred to another London hospital where I was once again given extensive tests. Finally I was told the results by the consultant, who in the presence of a number of students said "You have burnt out Ménière's disease. There is no cure for Ménière's disease but it does burn itself out. It does not usually recur but seems to have done so in your case!" He prescribed Stemetil tablets.

I had noticed that the attacks definitely seemed connected to the stress factor of my job. I was initially on three Stemetil a day, but managed to cut them down and avoided stressful situations whenever possible. It worked well and I usually managed to control the symptoms.

The good news is that since I retired and came to live in Norfolk I have not had one dizzy spell. I am extremely happy and sure that my contented emotional state contributes to the present stable period which I hope will last forever. I have no hearing in my right ear and have a hearing aid for the left. I just hope it doesn't deteriorate any further.

I would like other sufferers to know that there is hope of the symptoms ceasing for long periods. In my case I am convinced that keeping anxiety to a minimum is a major factor in the lessening of attacks.

'THE MENIERE'S TRAVELLER'

by

John Myall

Chobham, Surrey.

If ever there is a slot in the "Guinness Book of Records" for Ménière's attacks in the most exotic places, I am going to propose myself.

My world has spun amongst the ice-floes off Greenland, the bush of East Africa and even outside one of those naughty places in Bangkok. In case anyone gets the wrong idea, this last mentioned attack was not brought on by excitement or anticipation, - I was not on my way in at the time!!

Of one thing I am certain, the comfort and privacy of home is best.

Determination, fired by the needs of business (and a touch of wanderlust) kept me on the move and pushed wisdom to one side, - in spite of repeated discomfort, embarrassment and even personal danger. If more proof were needed that I was a glutton for punishment, I usually travelled alone.

My Ménière's first struck at the tender age of 38, although it must have been building up for some years as I had been a bit deaf in one ear for some time prior to its onset.

I awoke in the middle of the night after one those frightening nightmares when everything is spinning around. I was relieved to wake up, except the spinning hadn't stopped. I was promptly sick and my wife phoned the doctor. When he eventually arrived the worst was over and he suggested it was food poisoning.

The attacks returned during the following weeks and months with equal severity, usually without warning. The hospital specialist at first refused to believe that it could be Ménière's as diarrhoea had invariably accompanied my other troubles during the earlier attacks. "Diarrhoea is not a recognised symptom of Ménière's disease" he stated. "Maybe not, but it is a symptom of sheer terror", I replied. The learned physician had no doubt never experienced the joys of clinging to swaying walls and stumbling to a moving toilet, then making a split second decision as to which end was directed at the pan first!

As the varied selection of pills were having no effect, he agreed to do the "destruction job" operation, which cost me my hearing in that ear, and for one year life was bliss - until the other side started up.

Initially I was in despair as the nightmare I thought was over had now come back, and this time there could be no operation as I had to hang on to my remaining precious hearing for as long as possible. At least the dizziness didn't seem to be quite as bad this time round, or possibly I was just learning to cope better.

I tried any and every "alternative" treatment we could think of. During one bad spell I went to a faith healer in London. Two weeks after my first visit, the head cleared, the hearing improved and I was on top of the world. I continued to visit this lady every three or four weeks, in fact I was "hooked" on her, fearing that if I no longer went the problems would return. The bliss lasted for ten months, then for no reason back to misery. Maybe her powers only entitled her to give relief for a limited duration, or perhaps I was just in remission, I gave up going.

I was once treated by a Burmese doctor with acupuncture. On several occasions I even "got the needles" during an attack. With regularity, two hours after he finished the head would show an improvement and so would the hearing, but it never lasted for more than twenty four hours.

I had for many years run a wholesale fish company in London's West End, it was financially rewarding but the worries and pressure of work were enormous, so rightly or wrongly to this day I feel the stress involved caused the damage.

The travelling and the high pressure job were somewhat unfair on my family in many ways, and my wife was greatly relieved when the Ménière's forced me to sell up and slow down. Even daily commuting to London had been an ordeal, and she would never know how or when I would return home. On one occasion I was brought back in one of the firm's delivery vans, and spent the whole journey holding my head on with both hands, I really thought it was going to fall off. The selling up had another malicious twist of fate to it, as a few years previously a co-director, a cousin fact, had been forced out with Multiple Sclerosis, another dreadful nerve related illness of unknown cause that began with the letter "M".

I spent one year at home (we had recently moved to a smaller house), painting, decorating, gardening and idling away my time and the Ménière's disappeared, I thought, "What a wonderful world".

Feeling certain that getting rid of the stress, the Ménière's had cured itself, I started work again, this time in partnership in a gunsmiths. The pace of life was a lot more leisurely, and once again was the need for travel, but I enjoyed these trips anyway.

Then came the bomb-shell, the Ménière's had not cured itself, and initially it came back with a vengeance. Although stress was no longer on my daily menu, the damage had been done years back.

The attacks eventually diminished to a more manageable level of discomfort and of shorter duration, but the tinnitus and deafness increased alarmingly. The regular jet turbines screaming inside the skull were bad but the blurring of conversation seemed worse.

Having struggled to carry on it spite of "throwing a wobbly" from time to time, I felt as if I had won a small victory over "it". Now a new battle was starting, being in a world where the sounds that I received had less meaning to reality. A noise in the garden and I would ask my wife, "Is that a car or an aeroplane?" "Neither, it's next door's lawn-mower". With one ear dead I have no sense of sound direction either. Conversation is limited to quiet situations only, and even then with a degree of difficulty. Somehow me and lip-reading never quite made it together.

The hearing impairment forced me to sell my partnership in the gun trade.

I still have cause to travel and again this is usually alone, my wife doesn't like long distance flights, but deafness as opposed to the "wobblies" is a "whole different ball-game" as our transatlantic cousins would say. Getting about is comparatively easy as long as all goes according to plan, - then the fun really starts! I have been on the wrong plane in Iceland, the wrong hotel coach in Antigua, the wrong train in Italy and even the wrong bus in Basingstoke. Correct indicator boards and timetables are a Godsend, and British Rail does not have a monopoly on personnel who when asked "Does this train/boat/bus go to ......" Reply: "Grrhumffizz".

This could be positive, negative, or “My chewing gum has wrapped itself round my dentures”.

At home, early rising in the morning presents no problem, hearing wives have a use, they hear the alarm clock and give a sharp nudge. For the deaf lonesome traveller a different situation arises. Recently at a hotel in India I had to get up at 2am to get to Delhi airport for the early morning British Airways flight to Heathrow. I have in the past tried an alarm clock with a flashing light, it worked fine but not for the likes of me who habitually sleep face down and half buried under the pillow. My usual alarm has a vibrating box which is placed under the sheets or pillow, and is attached to the clock by a wire. The particular bed I was in was King sized (or possibly Rajah sized) and in such an enormous expanse I knew I would wander. It was a fair bet that come waking up time I would be a yard or more away from the machine which would then go on rattling unnoticed forever.

I had a brain-wave, it proved to be uncomfortable but it worked, I put the box down my pyjama trouser leg. On relating this incident to a friend, he said “I suppose you awoke to what could be called a deaf man’s thrill!”

It is now thirteen years since my world first spun out of control, and over a year since the last attack, although the balance is a little uncertain at times, particularly in the dark. I now work as a free-lance writer and as Tea Boy in the Ménière’s Society office in Woking. We live five miles away from the office alongside Chobham Common which is additionally handy for long walks so that the dog and I can put our literary thoughts in order. My hearing still just about lives on, and I regularly attend the local clay pigeon shoot of which I am secretary. (Rumour has it that they only keep me on in this capacity as I am the only one who can do joined up writing!) The sound of the guns is the only music my ear receives now.

I smoke, drink and readily munch my way through anything and everything that the health food faddists don't approve of. .... AND WHY NOT? I'VE SERVED MY TIME IN HELL ....

'THE OTHER SIDE'

by

Maureen Sheppard

Balham, London.

In 1983 Terry had not been feeling too good for a couple of weeks. He was 39, I was 37, we had three young children aged 11, 10 and 3. In the same year he was diagnosed as having Ménière's disease. When, after a few weeks it finally hit me, what this meant to us as a family, inevitable unemployment; financial hardship; no car which in turn meant no holidays as we go camping, but also Terry being at home all day - this may seem hard and hurtful on my part - I work evenings as a Youth & Community Worker so I valued my time during the day. For about a year we tried to carry on as normal, Terry was still employed, 'just', his credibility was running out as he spent more time out of work than in.

As mentioned, I'm a Youth & Community Worker, which I love. I see lots of problems which I can safely say I handle well, but that's outside my family life, my own I didn't handle very well. I didn't want to face up to it. When Terry got up in the mornings I would say over and over again to myself, 'He's feeling fine, he'll be OK for work, Please don't let him come staggering back having vomited and not able to go to work. I would say "Take a tablet and sleep a couple of hours, I'm sure you'll be all right, just a little bit late for work!" I wouldn't let myself think what Terry must be going through. Selfish? yes! but this was my survival kit.

Although in a bad way, Terry managed to keep an appointment at the hospital, the Hearing Therapist was shocked to see such a change in him. Although she recommended Terry stay at hospital he preferred to go home. However, she insisted that he at least went home by taxi and certainly not continue on to work. While Terry was making his way home, she rang to tell me what was happening, and in her own words said “In the 3 months since I last saw your husband, he’s gone from a healthy looking man to someone looking very ill” and to see him staggering along the corridor in the hospital, holding onto the walls had upset her. She went on to say about her concern regarding Terry’s employment, it was putting so much pressure on him, which in turn caused so many attacks. It was then it dawned on me the pressure I also was putting on him to keep a job - that was the turning point - there was no point in Terry suffering because of family commitments, and myself becoming a nervous wreck. Yes, there would be hardships, but with honesty and understanding on the part of us and the children as well, we could make it.

Looking back now over eight years, so many positive things have happened, only a few negative. It’s very true the saying ‘You find out who your true friends are in times of trouble’, yes, we’ve lost some so called friends, it’s strange even in this day and age the stigma that’s attached to unemployment. Oh yes, they are gradually phoning again since Terry has been employed by the Society - but they know where they can go! Our daughter Amanda was devastated when she had to give up her horse. The cost of keeping a horse stabled in London was out of our reach. Also trying to make two young teenagers aware of noise - record players on loud! “It hurts daddy’s ears”, “Why? he can’t hear well”, their friends popping in, “sorry they can’t any more, daddy’s in bed not well, he need’s peace and quiet”. Oh, you know the things that young teenagers and a five year old demand, but they did gradually get used to it, and proud parents we are, the way they turned out. I would like to think being aware of peoples disabilities has played a big part in this.

In 1985 Terry ran the "Ménière's Group" from home. What began as a small group escalated to over 1,000 members in less than three years. We had people in to help us now and then, but I must give special thanks to Eileen Little who came every week and helped us in so many ways. It was hard work but very rewarding. I know lots of Ménière's sufferers say "just to speak to another sufferer is such a relief", but as a non-sufferer, I gained so much knowledge from those who rang us.

Just imagine the Ménière's Society (re-named from 'Group') running from your home - meals eaten on laps, table now caters for typewriter, files, pens etc. Hall has boxes of stationery, kitchen wall had a large map dotted with pins where sufferers live, sitting-room housed the photo-copier. To be quite honest, I don't think there was a space left that didn't house something "Ménière's". Even the cat had her basket moved.

When the Society moved to Woking, it seemed strange having the house to ourselves again, it suddenly appeared much larger than it really was, even the cat didn't want to go back to her original place. She was much happier with her basket placed on the boxes of stationery, after all it's much warmer. Well tough luck "pussy cat", rewarding and enjoyable though it was, the equipment and stationery are now housed at Woking, Ah!!!!

CHAPTER FOUR

POET'S CORNER

'MY FIRST DATE'

by

Mrs. Y.M.

Newbury, Berks.

An invitation to tea,
I accepted happily,
The boy was good looking,
His mother was kind,
Although I was nervous
There was nothing on my mind
To suggest that disaster was looming.

The table was laid
With cakes all home-made,
Much laughter there was between us;
When suddenly my chair
Felt as if it wasn't there
And the room started spinning and zooming.

Oh no, not today,
It would mean I couldn't stay,
I was desperate to leave the table.
I must make for the loo
This I certainly knew
But I felt I wasn't able.

Oh the desire to let myself fall
To press my back against the wall
To feel the firmness and know I'm not spinning.
I was fighting a battle
And definitely not winning.

I thought the time had surely come
To tell my friends I had to go home,
All I could think of was my bed
Somewhere quiet to rest my head.
Both were staring at my ashen face
My fingers sought to find a place
To hold on firmly and try to stand,
They kindly helped and held my hand.

Their bewildered looks, - they couldn't quite grasp,
Why it had happened oh so fast.
To me it seemed like a big disaster
With the room spinning ever faster.
My boyfriend bundled me into his car
Thank goodness my home wasn't very far.
With relief on his face he made it quite plain
Not to expect to see him again.

I knew I shouldn't make a fuss,
I could have fallen under a bus.
I had to learn to live each day
To do life's bidding and not give way.
It was so much simpler to stay at home,
To write a letter or use the phone
Perhaps when I'm old I will think fate less mean,
I can't at the moment, NOT AT SIXTEEN.

'MY CONSTANT COMPANION'

by

Mrs. H.D.

Bundaberg, Queensland, Australia.

1. I have a constant companion; it's with me every minute;
You cannot see it you cannot hear it - you may think there's nothing in it.
2. But to me it is very real, and a lot of people have this;
It is noises in the head and its real name is "Tinnitus".
3. I had to learn to live with it and accept that it is mine;
(What else could I do?) even though it is hard at times.
4. "My Little Orchestra" I call it, to make it more acceptable;
The occasional tinkle of a Bellbird makes it more pleasurable.
5. A rippling stream is nice to hear, so is gentle rain as it falls;
But always, always the screeching cicadas are a continual background to it all.
6. My constant companion, my "Little Orchestra", what would I do without you?
No noises in my head; oh! what a relief, but maybe I would really miss you!!!!!

'ODE TO HYDROPS'

by

Mr.H.M. FRCS.

Gorleston, Norfolk.

The hour was late, the screen was dead
"Wake up my dear, it's time for bed"
She ope'd an eye and weakly spake
"I do not sleep, I am awake"
And then dropped off again.

He tottered out and once more tried
"Art up my love" and she replied
"No - but will be soon"
And then succumbed to further swoon.

At length she rose - a glass to fill
and find the morning Stemetil
And to her weary husband said
"Go - put these two beside the bed"
At last he lay down by her side
"Wake up! I cannot sleep she cried.

'MY PLEA'

by

Mrs. H.D.

Bundaberg, Queensland, Australia.

I am wandering everywhere, searching for a home,
may I please come in and with you make my home?
A little while may be all that I'll stay,
but then again I may never want to go away;
I know I can be quite unbearable that's true,
but I only want to be a friend with you.
You may not want to be a friend of mine,
but I promise I will try to be very kind.

Just listen to me and talk to me, and if you
must you can even be angry with me.
When you are busy you may not hear me at all.
Accept me if you can, then I'll be easier to ignore.
I promise I will not hurt you in any way,
although to you I may be a nuisance and in the way
When you are trying to hear what people are saying, and you
cannot understand for the noise I am making.
My name? Oh sorry, I forgot to give you my name.
I am called Tinnitus but I am not to blame.
For the distress I cause in some peoples lives,
when the noises I make sound like great bee hives.
Rushing water or rain falling into kegs,
hissing steam, clicking of grasshoppers legs;
The screeching of cicadas ever reaching for the sky,
but for all that, I am not really hurting you am I?

Now won't you please give me a home in your head?
I promise I'll be quiet when you're asleep in bed;
I feel so unloved, so unwanted and so sad,

but surely I am not all that bad.
I do make nice bearable sounds if you care to listen,
I will try to please you with everything in reason.
So I plead with you to please allow me to stay,
no one else wants me: please don't you send me away.

'Why?'

by

Mrs. M.C.

Stevenage, Herts.

Why does it happen to me
in the middle of Sunday tea?
Or in the middle of the night?
And why do I always fall to the right?

Why do I miss the start of what people say?
I'm not deaf every day.
I'm not really deaf at all,
and I really am not drunk when I fall.

I can swish around and be OK.
I can have a really hectic day,
then whilst sitting watching TV.
the world spins around violently.

Why do I suffer I really don't know,
sometimes it makes me feel so low.
Then I tell myself I could suffer from worse,
I still manage to continue my job as a nurse.

Oh no! here we go again,
sorry dear to be such a pain,
just ignore me,
let me be,
until I feel myself again.

'ODE TO A FELLOW SUFFERER'

by

Mrs. I.N.

Woodford Green, Essex.

Thank Heaven I'm feeling much better today,
the attacks of Ménière's have faded away.
No more vertigo I'm back on the beam,
the tinnitus is quiet it's been a bad dream.
I'm sitting in my garden relaxing in the sun,
It's good to be alive the battle has been won.
There's no-one around I'm here all alone,
It's pleasant and peaceful but there goes the phone.
Who can it be at this time of day,
most of my friends have all gone away.
Maybe it's Jill or Marlene or Sue,
but really I hope it just might be you.
It's such a long time since last we met,
Is it months or years I'm afraid I forget.
There's no time like the present so they say,
so do come and see me and make my day.
I'm not getting younger I'm now 79,
life is so short I'm near the end of the line.
But God willing whose blessings are manifold,
I hope I'm still here when I'm 100 years old.
And if those precious years are granted to me,
I earnestly pray they will be Ménière's free.

'ADVICE'

by

Mrs. I.N.

Woodford Green, Essex.

When you are having an attack of Ménière,
do not be afraid and do not despair.
Soon you will be as right as rain,
feeling like your old self again.
God has got His eye on you,
have faith and He will see you through.
So count your blessings when you're feeling blue,
there is someone out there much worse off than you.

* * *

'SLIMMING'

by

Mrs. D.F.

Bristol, Avon.

I don't waste money on slimming aids,
although at times I become quite fat;
After three months of whizzing and whirling around my figure is quite demure,
but please someone somewhere
'Find a Cure'!!!!!

'BLESSED ARE THEY'

by

Mrs. H.D.

Bundaberg, Queensland, Australia.

BLESSED ARE THEY - who gain my attention, face me and speak clearly, to help avoid a wrong interpretation.
BLESSED ARE THEY - Who have patience with me when I am unable to follow the conversation, especially in a crowd or a noisy situation.
BLESSED ARE THEY - Who realise that when I do not answer at once, I have not heard or am trying to establish what has been said.
BLESSED ARE THEY - Who understand that because of my hearing disability and my impaired eye-sight, my mind tends to be a little slow in comprehension.
BLESSED ARE THEY - Who can realise how hard it is for me to grasp what is being said, when they themselves can hear every word clearly.
BLESSED ARE THEY - Who encourage me to keep on trying to learn to speech-read, when I feel I just want to quit.
BLESSED ARE THEY - Who never ever say "It doesn't matter" and turn away. To me, it really does matter, very much.
BLESSED ARE THEY - Who encourage me to be outgoing rather than withdrawing from society - because of the fear of embarrassment to others and to myself.
BLESSED ARE THEY - Who hears my cries of frustration and loneliness and support me with love and compassion to accept and try to overcome my disabilities.
BLESSED ARE THEY INDEED, WHO ACCEPT ME JUST AS I AM.

"Better Hearing" June,1989

'A TALE OF MENIERE'S'

by

Mrs. P.N.

Wimborne, Dorset.

Twenty three years ago this year,
I had an odd feeling in my ear.
The world whirled round, I felt so low,
the doctor said "It's vertigo".
"Ménière's disease is what you've got,
I'm afraid yours is an unhappy lot".

I crawled upstairs on hands and knees,
my state of health just did not please.
My family wondered just what to do,
"Come on mum, this is not like you".

The years rolled by and various pills
were taken down to soothe my ills,
but life became a precarious thing
of ups and downs, and my ears started to sing.

Hearing slowly faded out
and family had to start to shout,
outside sounds became quite mute,
but in my ears noise is acute!

So now I must soldier on,
revived by Serc and Stemetil.
A gallant husband is my strength
and helps to fortify my will.

So all in all it's not so bad,
and there are days that make one glad.
There may be times that make one curse,
but there are things so very much worse.

Now I've reached three score and ten
I'm still an active Septuagenarian!
I stay on my feet - though now and then
I confess the world goes in a spin.

* * *

'YOU'VE GOT TO LEARN TO LIVE WITH IT'

by

Terry Sheppard

Balham, London.

Now here's a little story, you'll want to read to the end.
But if you've not heard of Ménière's disease, you could get bored my friend.

It all begins with a buzzing, a ringing or a hiss.
The volume goes up on the telly, with the odd word often amiss.

Then the fretful day arrives, when the world starts spinning round,
so much before you notice, you are falling to the ground.

The doctor says 'I'm not quite sure' and says 'You need a test'.
The appointment is made, for nine months time, meantime one copes as one knows best.

When given time to think of it, the mind plays funny tricks.
One starts to think of tumours, it tallies with the 'fits'.

They say you need a scan of sorts, confirming your inner fears.
The lack of reassurance, often results in a flood of tears.

Hearing; blood, and other tests, hope there aren't many more,
I didn't like the water one, I nearly fell to the floor.

'It could be a syndrome called Ménière's disease, a condition of the inner ear,
Vertigo, Tinnitus, Deafness .... Nothing to Fear!'

'You've got to learn to Live with it' and quoting from well rehearsed text,
'Reduce your fluids, caffeine and salt, stop smoking, drinking...... NEXT'.

I found I was out in the street again, without saying, 'But which way and why!
I've never heard of, what did he call it, am I going to die?

All this was written some time ago and I have discovered how to cope,
I'll not make light of Ménière's disease but no matter what

THERE'S ALWAYS ROOM FOR HOPE.

'FOOTSTEPS'

by

Mrs. S.M.

Burton-on-Trent, Staffs.

Footsteps behind me how hollow they sound,
just like a jack hammer hitting the ground,
I pause by a window and peer within,
my ears are aching, my heads in a spin.

Footsteps have gone now, noise fades away,
but my head is pounding as I start to sway,
people brush passed me, I know what they think,
just another - had too much to drink!

Footsteps around me, such noise, such speed,
will no-one provide me the help that I need?
I find my card - just read it - PLEASE?
Do I have to grovel on bended knees?

Footsteps approach, much softer, how kind,
and soon the noise is left far behind,
I thank the footsteps for being aware,
It's nice to know that someone DOES care!

'TOWARDS THE DAWN'

by

(Anon)

An Ode written by a member which gives her great comfort when she recites it to herself during the bad spells - she hopes it may also help others in hours of need.

Be brave when dark clouds dim your path,
Be strong when hope and faith seem past.
Look for the light to show the way,
Look for the dawn of another day.

Don't hide the grief that's in your heart,
There's always a friend to take a part
-- in showing you faith can again be born --

'IT'S ONLY TINNITUS'

by

Mrs. Y.M.

Newbury, Berks.

A noise in the ear 'That's nothing' they cry, don't make a fuss,
Just ignore it - it may go away, It's only Tinnitus

You can't sleep at night, it give you bad dreams,
'Oh, don't keep telling us',
Turn on the radio, bury your head
It's only Tinnitus.

Of course you're not mad, who said you were?
It certainly wasn't us.
Now would we laugh, be so unkind?
It's only Tinnitus.

A trip to the Doc, for comfort I guess,
my problem to discuss,
'Just take these pills' he gaily cries
'It's only Tinnitus'.

'SILENCE IN THE LIBRARY'

by

Mr. H.F.

Belfast, N.Ireland.

I have these noises, you see,
Yes, inside of me.
No, they cause me no pain,
well, I suppose, but let me explain.
In each ear I have these noises, very loud at times you know,
although really I suppose you wouldn't know.
What sort of noise did you say?
It's the noises make me hear that way,
yes, I get them every day.
No, they never go away.
It's part of a disease,
No, it's not contagious, please
I like to talk about it.
Now let me explain these noises, yes at times they're bad,
they sometimes nearly drive me mad,
Yes, I suppose it is very sad.
During the day I get some peace,
No, I'm not saying that they cease
you know what I mean, other sounds you see
make it easier for me.
At night when I lie in bed
the noises pounding in my head,
- What's that you said?
Well, yes it is annoying, nice to have talked to you -
Do you fancy a beer?
quiet in here.
Yes, quieter for you than for me,
you've picked your books I see.
Could you wait till I pay my fine,

and do you see that 'silence' sign?
Now that's what I yearn for all the time!

* * *

'LEAVING HOSPITAL'

by

Mrs. Y.M.

Newbury, Berks.

With giddy attacks every two or three weeks
an operation had seemed the answer,
After which, learning to walk and feeding myself was an all time job to master.

At first I couldn't find my mouth
but solved this pretty soon,
If I didn't want to starve to death
I had to take it to the spoon.

Walking was the hardest bit,
I clung like mad to my bed
with one nurse holding onto my arm
and another steadying my head.

First one foot forward then the other,
everything seemed to be moving too,
how to turn round when I got to the end?
I really didn't have a clue.

The whole ward clapped and cheered
as I made my way back into bed,
'That feels better I know' said the nurse,
I couldn't tell her I felt nearly dead.

The patients were of varying ages,
though they all seemed younger than me,
'Well done' cried my neighbour -
'You did very well' - and she was only three!

Next day the surgeon arrived
to see what progress I'd made,
In his hand was a five pound note,
I should think he'd just been paid.

If you pick this up without falling,
you can pack your bags today.
Quick as a flash I scooped it up
while he looked on in dismay.

He obviously wasn't expecting this
but a promise is a promise they say;
Although everything was still spinning about
I didn't intend to stay another day.

From then on all was bustle
to leave as fast as I could,
I didn't even stop to dress
although I knew I really should.

I knew I must start as I meant to go on,
so tackled the stairs on my own;
my parents went down before me
and didn't hear my desolate groan.

I will never forget that journey
one step at a time did I take,
It's one thing to tell your body to do
and another thing to make.

CHAPTER FIVE

BIBS N' BOBS

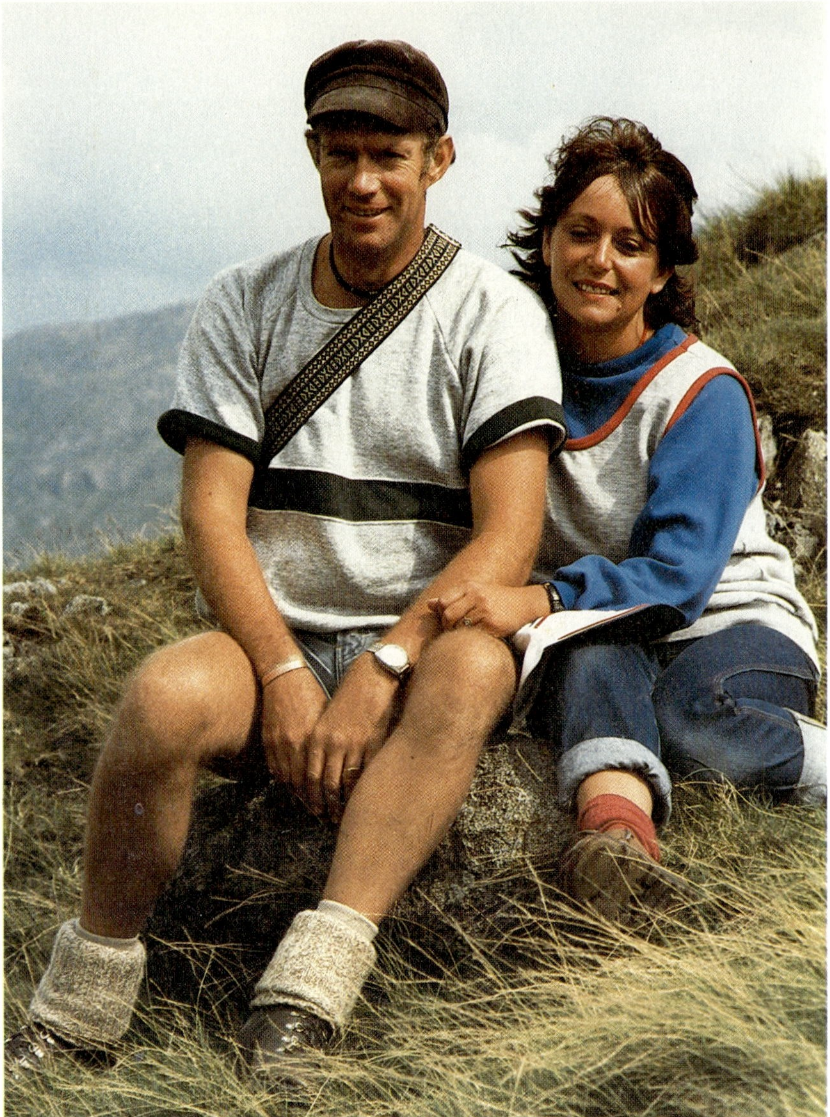

Terry, with his wife Maureen, still enjoy fell walking, seen here on Harter Fell, Cumbria.

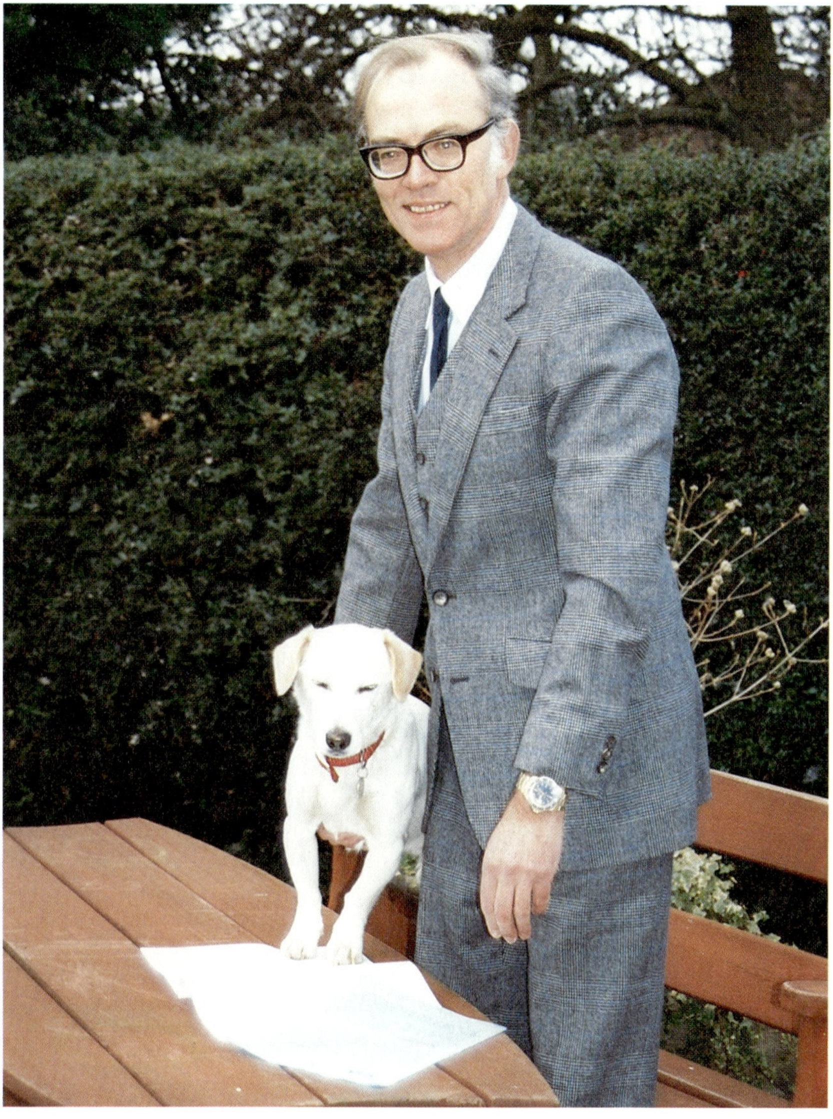

John Myall, editor of 'Spin', the Ménière's Society newsletter, discusses the next publication with Max, his assistant.

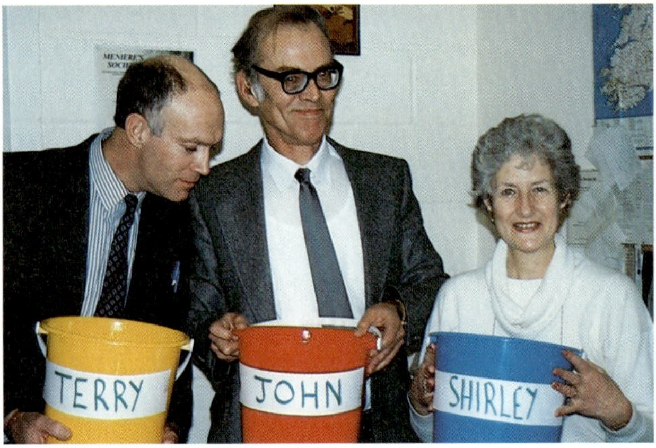

Ménière's sufferers do possess a sense of humour. Co-Ordinator Terry, with volunteers John and Shirley have personalised buckets at the ready - just in case....

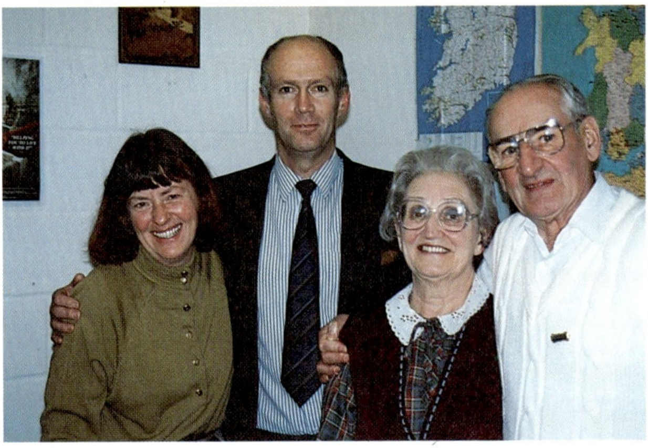

Contact with overseas groups is always welcome. From left to right, Vivien Barton from Ménière's Australia, with Terry, Marie and husband Gordon, at the Woking office.

'ELECTRICAL MENIERE'S.......?'

by

Mr. J.F.

Barnet, Herts.

I think it was Swift who wrote a pamphlet called "The World Turned Up-side-down". It did so for me on a wartime site near Guildford circa 1940.

Being in a mobile anti-aircraft unit we were used to being moved about, and were usually only allowed a couple of hours to pack up and go.

On one particular occasion after we had received our "marching orders" we were as usual running around packing things up. There was an electrical feed cable running from the guard-house near the gate to a command post, and I was very concerned about retrieving this particular item that I had 'rescued' from another unit's site. I sent my assistant to the guard-house to pull out the fuses. This was a good 100 yards away. I stood at the command post waiting to cut the cable when I saw him emerge from the guard-house door, and I thought he said OK.

I made the cut and was immediately held in a vice-like clamp as my muscles reacted to the electricity coursing through them. My brain was whirling round and the sound in my ears was a whoosh, whoosh, - presumably at 50 hertz a second!

How long this persisted I don't know, but I remember thinking I must call for help. Eventually I collapsed, but when pulled up by a couple of squaddies, recovered swiftly and in five minutes was rushing around again.

The world still revolves round me now and again when I have an attack, and I do sometimes wonder if this former incident had anything to do with it? - But then it was nearly 50 years ago.

* * *

'AT WORK'

by

Mrs. P.V.

Crowborough, East Sussex.

I work for a very understanding boss who, despite the fact that he really thought my attacks were due to an over-indulgence of the gin bottle, realised that when I went missing for long periods, that I was in all probability, either with my head down the toilet or lying on the floor. Now the only suitable floor to lie on was the one in the Board Room which, in addition to the coat stand also had a T-shaped table in it and I used to lie parallel to the head of the T, - furthest from the door and out of sight to anyone entering.

One particular day I was recovering from an attack during working hours by lying on the floor covered with coats when the door opened and into the Board Room came another Director, a Department Manager, and a prospective applicant for a senior position within the company.

What a dilemma I was in......should I lay there and hope no-one would notice or should I stand up (if I could) and get out......I decided on the latter and by raising myself onto my knees and by gripping the edge of the Board Room table, shuffled to the nearest radiator which I hung onto like grim death until I was able to haul myself up and edge along the wall, - which unfortunately kept moving. This took some minutes to accomplish during which time all three stood rooted to the ground and my lasting impression of this encounter was of three men staring boggle eyed at this shuffling, tottering dishevelled female who was muttering "I really must take more water with it next time"........

Needless to say from that day to this a cursory inspection of the Board Room is made before it is used.

* * *

'IF THE CAP FITS......'

by

(Anon)

A while back I was going through a phase of severe and frequent Ménière's attacks. During this time we had a clergyman staying with us overnight.

He rose in the morning after my husband had left for work, only to find me laid out with yet another attack, so he had to get his own breakfast.

Out of the kindness of his heart he decided this was the time to do his "God thing" on me before leaving. He proceeded to explain that my suffering was due to my way of life, my attitude to religion and a difficult marriage, (which after 30 years is still one of the best!) I'm sure he went on his way feeling much better.

But guess who, within a year, was diagnosed as having Ménière's....... And they say the wheels of God grind slowly!!! ....

'ME AND MENIERE'S'

by

Mrs. M.L.

Cirencester, Glos.

The place, the hotel boat "Tranquil Rose" moored at Stoke Bruerne on the Grand Union Canal. The date, 8th October, 1990, last day of a week's cruise.

That evening I and my fellow passengers were as happy as the Canterbury pilgrims were on their last day. Many tales had been told on the "Tranquil Rose" too during the week, in English, Canadian and American voices.

We had our last delicious dinner, ending with baked Alaska, (brought in flaming). As we went off to pack somebody said "The winds getting up".

It certainly was. In all my fifteen years of cruising on the canals I have never known anything like it. The wind roared, the "Tranquil Rose" rocked and so did I. I did not sleep and felt the night would never end.

At last, time to get up. But I couldn't raise my head. "This is it" I thought. "I've had it". I tried deep breathing and relaxation and at last could stagger to my feet. I was dizzy and felt sick and could not face breakfast.

When I got home I was still ill and the doctor came. "Ménière's disease" he said. "The storm?" I asked. "Oh no", he said. But I wonder, when I think of the tossing.

I have been ill off and on since then and decided to try relaxation, visualisation and affirmation. This was a great help and has kept Ménière's at bay since. If I feel dizzy when I wake up I lie down and do my relaxation exercises. Then I visualise my middle ears and say to them mentally "You are equally balanced. I am no longer feeling dizzy or sick". I repeat this several times. It is important to be positive. The effect is miraculous.

Soon I shall be off on my first cruise of 1991, on the upper reaches of the Thames. This is the perfect holiday for such as I. I can stay on board all the time, sitting out in the well deck for hours, getting lots of fresh air. Or I can go for a walk when the boat moors. Only about 8 passengers and a splendid crew who will look after me if I am not well. Lucky, lucky me!

* * *

'FROM A MENIERE'S SELF-HELP GROUP MEMBER'

by

Mr. K.P.N.

Leics.

I was pleasantly surprised when I read in our local paper that a Self-Help/Support Group of the National Ménière's Society was being formed in our area.

Having been hit by this devastating and unknown (to me) condition four months earlier, and having been off work all that time - I crawl around inspecting machinery and buildings and it's not the ideal job for a Ménière's sufferer - I had never met any other sufferers, and did not have any idea there was such a thing as a National Society.

We all met for the first time in someone's lounge, six of us, four sufferers and two helpers, and it was good to be able to talk over my experiences with people who really understood, and to hear their experiences also. Now, six months later, there are 12 of us, and we are hoping to form another group in our area soon. We meet once a month for the "business" meeting, though its hard to get a word in edgeways, sometimes, and in between we arrange a purely "social" meeting. Cream tea in someone's garden, we keep trying for, but usually the weather turns against us and we end up in the kitchen or conservatory scoffing toasted teacakes. We're also planning a visit to a garden centre - one where they have refreshments, of course! We are planning to have a go at some fund-raising for the main Society soon, but it's also a bit of an excuse to get together for a natter, if we're honest!

We all look forward to the meetings, and every one of our sufferers are convinced they feel better since meeting each other.

* * *

'THE PERILS OF WEETABIX?'

by

Mr. R.N. Silsden,

Yorks.

When I contracted Ménière's I had to stop working; being at home all day my weight ballooned up to 16 stone.

On one of my monthly visits to the doctor I mentioned this and he gave me a diet sheet, which started each day with a Weetabix. After two days of this I had the most surprising attacks, instead of things flying around in an anti-clockwise direction they fell from the ceiling to the floor.

I left them out for three days then tried again but it was the same result! On mentioning this to the doctor he said "Oh, it's the extra dairy produce, have you tried them with warm water?' Once again the result was another attack just like the others. Back to the doctor and this time he said 'It might be the Weetabix, try Shredded Wheat'.

I believe that if anything, Shredded Wheat and warm water is worse than Weetabix and warm water, and the result was the same, attacks with everything seeming to fall from the ceiling. 'You must have an allergy' he told me on my next visit.

Now I keep off all forms of wheat bran and those strange attacks never returned. I also keep off all citrus fruits, bacon, ham, dairy produce, coffee, shellfish and anything out of a tin, - but I still weigh 14 stone.

'A TIP FOR THE BED-BOUND'

by

Mr. J.S.

East Lothian.

Living on my own and with an upstairs bedroom, I was faced with the problem of how does the doctor get in if my good neighbour is away and the door is locked?

Solution: a length of string, long enough to reach from the bedroom window to ground level. One end has a heavy brass key ring with key attached, and the other is tied to a hook screwed into the skirting board.

Even during an attack I can manage to crawl from my bed with my eyes shut, open the window and toss the key out.

* * *

'IT HAPPENS TO THE BEST OF US'

by

Mrs. P.D.

I know the usual place one should use for heaving up, to put it politely, but I am sure many Ménière's sufferers have at times resorted to the oddest receptacle. Not that mine was all that odd, just the most practical at hand at that time, - it was a fancy plastic container for the office plant.

My husband had been called to collect me, and no way was I travelling home in a taxi without some sort of receptacle - much to my husband's embarrassment. Although on reflection it may have been a bigger embarrassment to the pocket if he had to pay for the cleaning of the taxi!

'THE GOOD SAMARITAN'

by

Mr. H.D.

It was in the early and dramatic stage of Ménière's with the dreadful spinning head and motion sickness that I started an attack on the way to work.

As I staggered helplessly about the pavement, I heard a passer-by loudly call out "How disgusting! and so early in the day". Later I found myself clinging to a railing and desperately wondering what to do. Suddenly a kindly voice said "Can I help? I live in the house opposite, would you like to come in and sit for a while?"

It was a lady who must have been watching my antics from her window. I gladly accepted her invitation and attempted to explain my problem and hastened to assure her that it was not caused by the demon drink.

The good lady helped me over the worst of the attack until I was able to phone a friend who collected me in a car.

That incident happened over twenty five years ago and my attacks have long since subsided, but I will always remember with gratitude that gesture of kindness from a total stranger.

'THE ONLY GOOD THING ABOUT MENIERE'S.....'?

by

Mrs. A.L.

Bilston, West Mids.

I have suffered from Ménière's for 25 years, and am now 66. The doctor tells me it won't kill me ..... but then it doesn't do me any good either!!

My husband says the good thing about the attacks is that we have plenty of food left. I agree that they certainly keep me slim.

* * *

'ANOTHER GOOD THING.....'

by

Mrs. H.B.

Bristol, Avon.

I never realised just how much my husband, children, sisters and friends loved me. I have always been fairly healthy during my life, but when my attacks started, the support and concern they showed, and have continued to do so, made me aware of how lucky I am. So good things do come out of bad sometimes.

'RANDOM THOUGHTS'

by

Mrs. D.M.

Willmington, Kent.

If I'm out with my family and Ménière's is mentioned, I am then ignored and people ask my husband "Can she hear? Can she talk?" As I am getting more confident with my lip-reading and am fortunate enough to have some hearing (with an aid), I answer for myself "I can only hear when aided by lip-reading, but by Golly can I talk!"

When I was much younger I envied other people in two things, the ability to ride a bicycle and to swim. I spent hours with my brothers trying to learn to ride, only to find that when they let go I was still pedalling like mad lying on on the ground getting nowhere fast. I stuck it for two years then gave up. I eventually learnt to drive a car but that beat me as the Ménière's increased, although at first I didn't know what it was.

As for swimming, I still go to the pool and try. My husband is very good he stays with me as I grip on the sides and kick my legs, - just in case I have an attack. So my two longed for ambitions are still beyond me.

I find Serc is a great help, and look forward to receiving the Society's newsletter, which keeps you in touch and lets you know you are not alone.

I'm fortunate in having a doctor whose mother is a sufferer, although I don't consider myself a sufferer as such - just incapacitated at times. I'm damned if "It" is going to rule my life. My doctor said I should not go out alone and should always take a stick, I guess I'm too pig-headed to do what I'm told.

I ran a cub scout pack for 14 years, but that became too much so I now run a Darby and Joan club instead, which although demanding isn't so physically exhausting.

I find escalators a pain and try to laugh as I try harder to keep my balance, lifts are easier as long as there is something solid to grab. Stairs can be a bind, lighthouses and ladders are beyond me so I avoid them like the plague.

Isn't it annoying when you are on the wrong side of a large room and can't go round the edge because of all the people. You either stagger across by yourself or ask for help. I usually find people are very kind and helpful.

Hearing is a problem, concentrating on lip-reading is tiring, but I find the classes are fun.

I suppose I'm an optimist, I always hope that I shall be given that inner strength to carry on, and most times I can even if I am seeing the world through a revolving door, and when there's a lull, well, that's a bonus.

'FINAL ACCOUNT'

by

Mr. A.W.

Willingham, Cambs.

I'm an accountant, and for many years I joked; "An old accountant never dies, he merely loses his balance". This has taken on a whole new meaning now that I have got M.D.!

When I went to see my doctor for the fourth time with vertigo, (before M.D. was diagnosed) he greeted me with, "Hello, and how is the world going round for you then!"

* * *

EXTRACTS FROM NEWSLETTERS...

'TERRY AT THE OFFICE'

People write or telephone asking a variety of questions. Many ask about problems arising from the loss of hearing and in particular about not hearing the door bell or television. Most people have heard of the induction loop system which is basically a wire surrounding the room, each end connected to an amplifier. When using a hearing aid switched to the 'T' position, sound from a microphone is fed directly into the aid. You can imagine my surprise when a caller who, judging age by her voice, was obviously past caring about birth control, asked for information on "how can I arrange to have a coil fitted".........

Another caller requested information regarding the avoidance of vomiting during an attack.

"Have you tried suppositories?" I asked.

"Are they the things you put in your ear?" she queried.

I was tempted to say "You could always try".

* * *

'FLYING WITH MENIERE'S'

We receive quite a few letters from sufferers wanting to plan a holiday abroad who are worried about the effects of flying. We have been advised that there is no medical evidence to show that a sufferer should not travel by air. However some people are naturally nervous of flying and any excitement or aggravation prior to or during the trip can cause tension. Stress most certainly can trigger an attack.

One precaution you can take is to inform your doctor beforehand in case there are other ear related problems.

As far as I can recall we have received no more than three letters from members who claim that the pressure change induced their attacks. Two referred to planes and the other to high mountains. On the other hand several have claimed that the plane trip improved things - if only temporarily.

I personally have spent many hundreds of hours in the air since the onset of Ménière's. Yes, I have had in-flight attacks but I put this down to the law of averages. I have had the "wobblies" in all sorts of odd places on earth so why not a couple up on the clouds, just for variety!

‘HOLIDAY INSURANCE’

When you take out medical or holiday insurance, do you carefully read through the policy? Up to date I have never bothered too much, but it has been pointed out to us that this onerous little task could be very important.

If the application form asks for details of any illnesses etc., you must disclose to them about your Ménière’s. Failure to do so could give them the excuse to wriggle out of payment should you have to make a claim.

* * *

‘MY HUSBAND’S WISDOM’

by

Mrs. M.J.

Brislington, Bristol.

One night I awoke and found myself making a ghastly noise while trying not to be sick, - I have chronic asthma and bronchitis as well as Ménière’s - and being sick when already short of breath is, to say the least, not very pleasant.

To my astonishment, my husband got out of bed, picked our peacefully sleeping cat from the bed, and marched out the room with him to put the bewildered animal outside.

Between gulps for air I asked “Why?”

“He was about to be sick” he replied, then got back into bed and went to sleep!

On another occasion I was shaking my head violently (very unwise) as a moth pitched on me, I tumbled across the room landing on both knees on the floor. My husband came in and solemnly said "You can say a prayer for me while you're down there" then got into bed and went to sleep quite oblivious that I had fallen.

When I had the worst bout of flu ever, with the complications of bronchitis and asthma, followed by severe Ménière's I was in bed for five months and lost over two stone in weight.

I had gone very deaf in the process, and my son sat on the edge of the bed and took hold of my hand. Expecting words of comfort (Ha! Ha!) he shouted "Mum you look worse than when I saw grandpa in hospital, and I thought he was dying". He then proceeded to give me details of a TV programme he had seen about embalming! My husband who was reading the evening paper, then loudly informed me that he had just seen that the price of funerals had gone up as well.

I must add that I am totally cared for when ill, but somehow men are different in their attitudes, but at least it provides a few laughs one way or another.

'THE CURE FOR MENIERE'S'

by

John Myall,

Chobham, Surrey.

The cure for Ménière's is to give up everything you enjoy doing! This is the way it seemed to me after years of varied advice from conventional and alternative medical practitioners.

Shortly after M.D. was first diagnosed I was referred to a hospital in London where a multitude of test were carried out. I also filled out an extensive questionnaire on hobbies, foods regularly eaten, drugs taken over the years, work and general lifestyle. The "eminent" consultant finally seized upon the fact that I did a lot of rifle shooting at Bisley and clay pigeon shooting. "You must give it up, the noise is probably the cause of your troubles". The faith in the diagnosis plummeted to zero as no-one had bothered to ask if I regularly wore any form of ear protection when shooting. I always do - the best you can get. As a consolation prize I was given a different bottle of pills as an alternative to my regular prescription. I had tried them before and they didn't do any good the first time either!

A further try with the conventional was yet another hospital in London, this time the idea was a virtual salt free diet with liquid intake severely curtailed. I managed to last out for six months. Goodbye to kippers, bacon and all the other foods of the gods. The meagre liquid intake somehow didn't leave room for the occasional morale boosting gin and tonic. Eggs, chips, spaghetti, they all tasted revolting, the Ménière's showed no sign of improvement; it was like lifting away a cloud of doom when I finally gave up.

The acupuncturist said "You must abstain from alcohol". Was this an excuse because his needles were not having the desired effect? Did he really believe his electrical stimuli were being drowned in a sea of booze? I could not accept that one or two daily drinks were the ruination of the treatment. Goodbye acupuncturist.

"Give up smoking" cried the multitude of self righteous. "Don't you know its bad for you, haven't you seen the overwhelming evidence against it?" "There was once overwhelming evidence to show the earth was flat" I replied; "Anyway I enjoy it". I did give up once, unfortunately this great effort coincided with one of my worst series of attacks ever. It probably was just that - coincidence, but there was a nagging thought "could it have been withdrawal symptoms livening things up a bit?" I gave up trying to give up.

"Have you ever considered a vegetarian diet?" asked the faith healer. "No, I have an on-going love affair with steak and kidney puddings" said I. "It would cleanse the system" persisted the healer. "I have a vegetarian colleague with Ménière's and he gets worse attacks than I do". I countered. Thus ended the topic of conversation. Personally I have never been convinced of the "If it hurts it must be doing you good" theory of medicine. However, I genuinely believe that some sufferers do get relief with special diets etc., I just don't happen to be one of them.

It is fourteen years since the first attacks, they are now infrequent and mild in comparison to the early days, although the balance is a bit shaky particularly in the dark. I no longer take any pills, something I have gladly given up. On the debit side my hearing is a mess. Even with a hearing aid, all sound is badly distorted.

However, I still go clay pigeon shooting, have my couple of daily tots and a contented puff of a cigarette. To my wife's envy I eat everything and anything without putting on any weight.

Would I have kept my sanity if I had given everything up?

Reproduced from Newsletter No.22

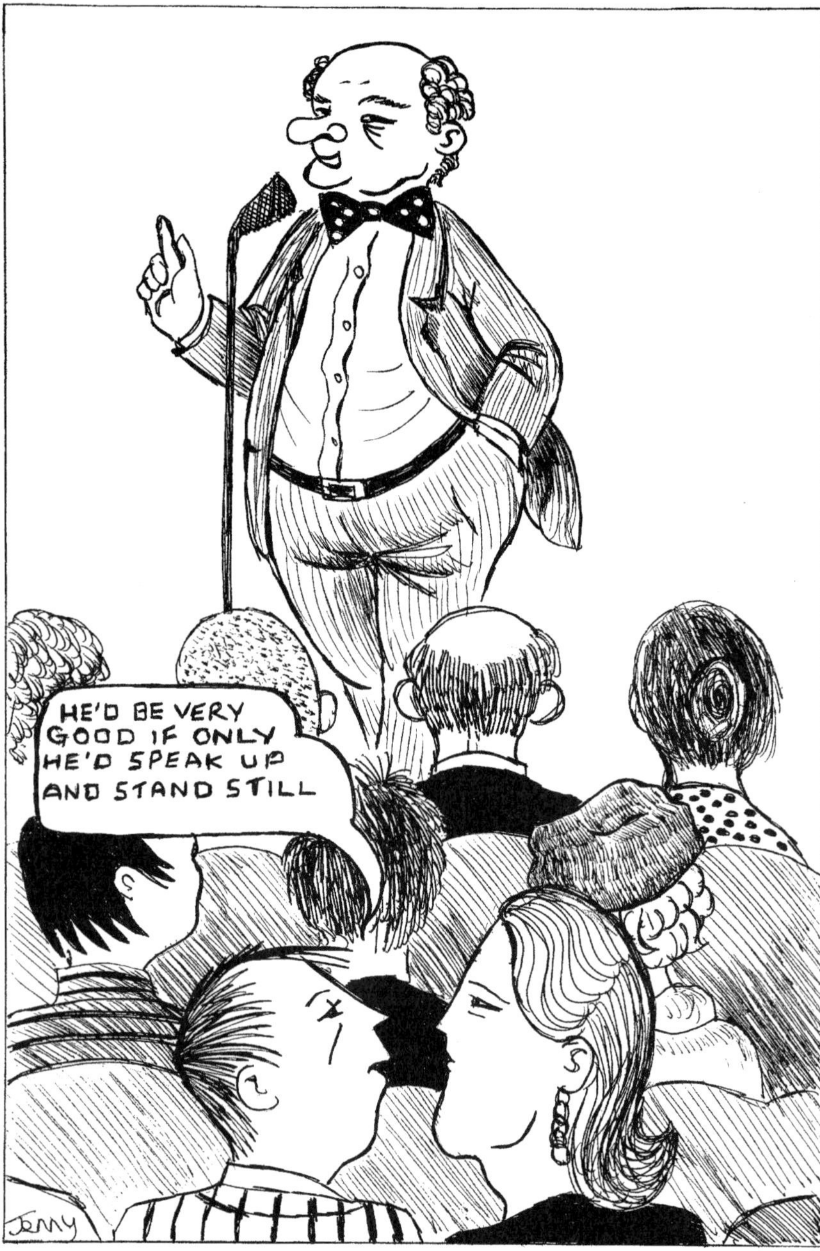
HE'D BE VERY GOOD IF ONLY HE'D SPEAK UP AND STAND STILL
JENNY

'BELLE VIEW HOUSE'

North Road, West Lodge, Cornwall. Tel. 05036 2935

by

David Winsper

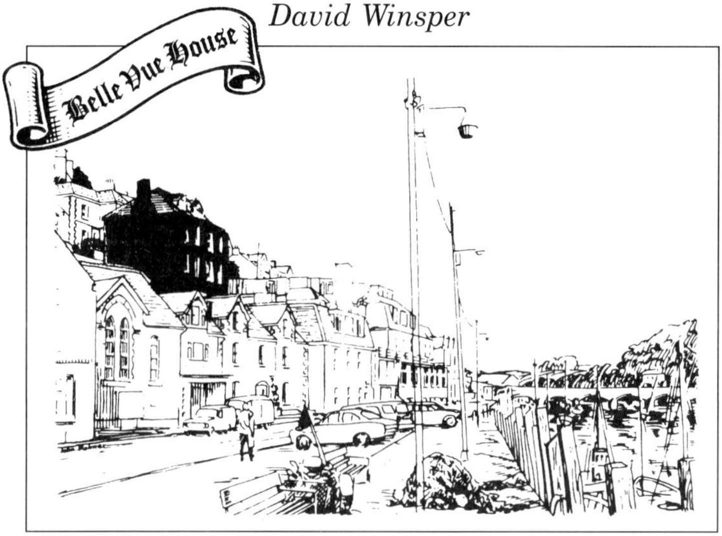

The guest house is run by David and Kate Winsper, and as David is himself a Ménière's sufferer they have first hand knowledge and understanding of the problems caused by the illness.. . .

Three years ago, Kate and I moved to Cornwall to run this large guest house. The idea was for a peaceful life with less stress to help me cope with my Ménière's condition, - some chance!! In that time we have had our fair share of knocks, but most of all we've had some good laughs.

'Belle Vue House' is enviably situated overlooking the quays of both East and West Looe with their never ending variety of sea and river traffic. Fishing boats discharging their catches are a favourite to young and old alike. The quaint towns and the immediate locality provide numerous activities such as fishing, golf, tennis, horse riding and bowls, whilst many excursions may be taken by land or sea to places of both natural or historic interest. There is a sandy beach ideal for children and providing safe bathing. The guest house is only two minutes from the shops of West Looe or the regular passenger ferries give ready access to East Looe. An excellent centre for the holidaymaker, the South Cornish coastline is an area of outstanding natural beauty with its many coves, inlets and beaches.

We hope to have many more Ménière's sufferers visit us where they will be assured of a kindly and understanding welcome.

* * *

'HELPFUL COLLEAGUES AT WORK'

by

John Myall

Chobham, Surrey.

After the initial onslaught of Ménière's, I was explaining to my Scottish accountant about the problems in the left ear causing a loss of balance. With his usual wicked sense of humour he advised: "Why do ye nae put a wee piece of lead in the other ear to balance things up? In your case the lead could be injected wi' a revolver!"

Several years later at another job I staggered to the storeroom out the back to 'enjoy' my attack of the wobbles in peace and quiet. My partner came in and said "Do you want me to call the doctor....... or the knacker's yard?"

CHAPTER SIX

ABOUT THE MENIERE'S SOCIETY

MENIERE'S SOCIETY©

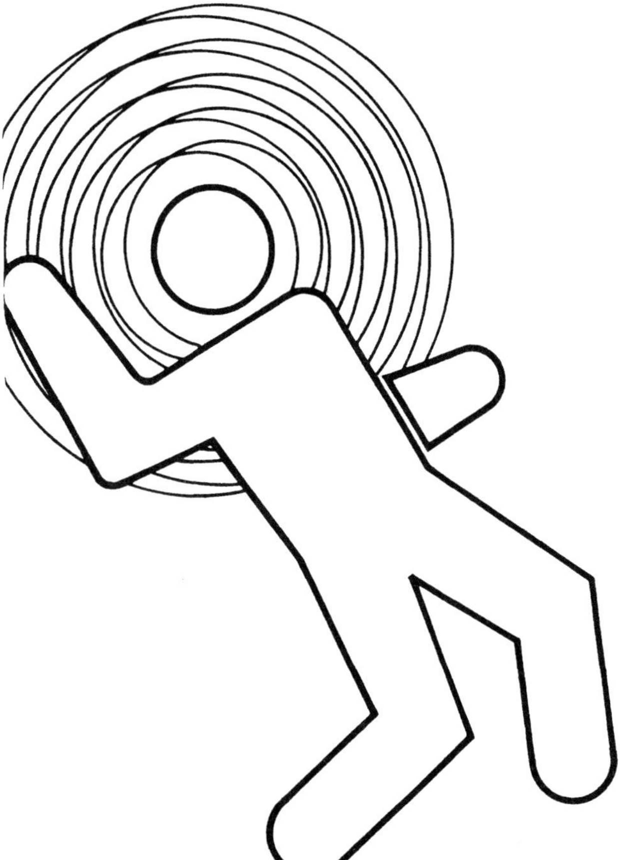

President & Founder
Mrs. Marie Nobbs MBE

Patrons
Lady Marjorie Clark
Mr. Ian Chapman CBE, FRCA, D.Lit.

Hon. Chairman
Miss Catrin Williams FRCS

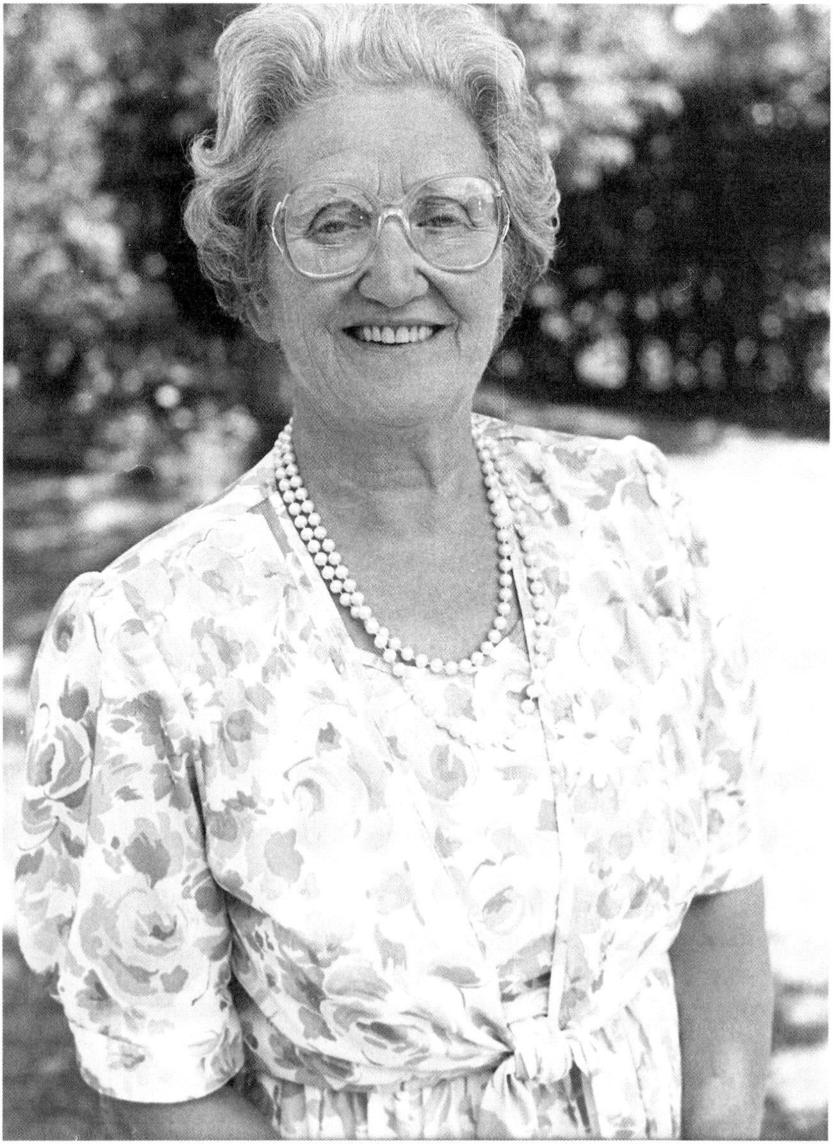

Marie B. Nobbs. MBE.
Life President and Founder of the Ménière's Society

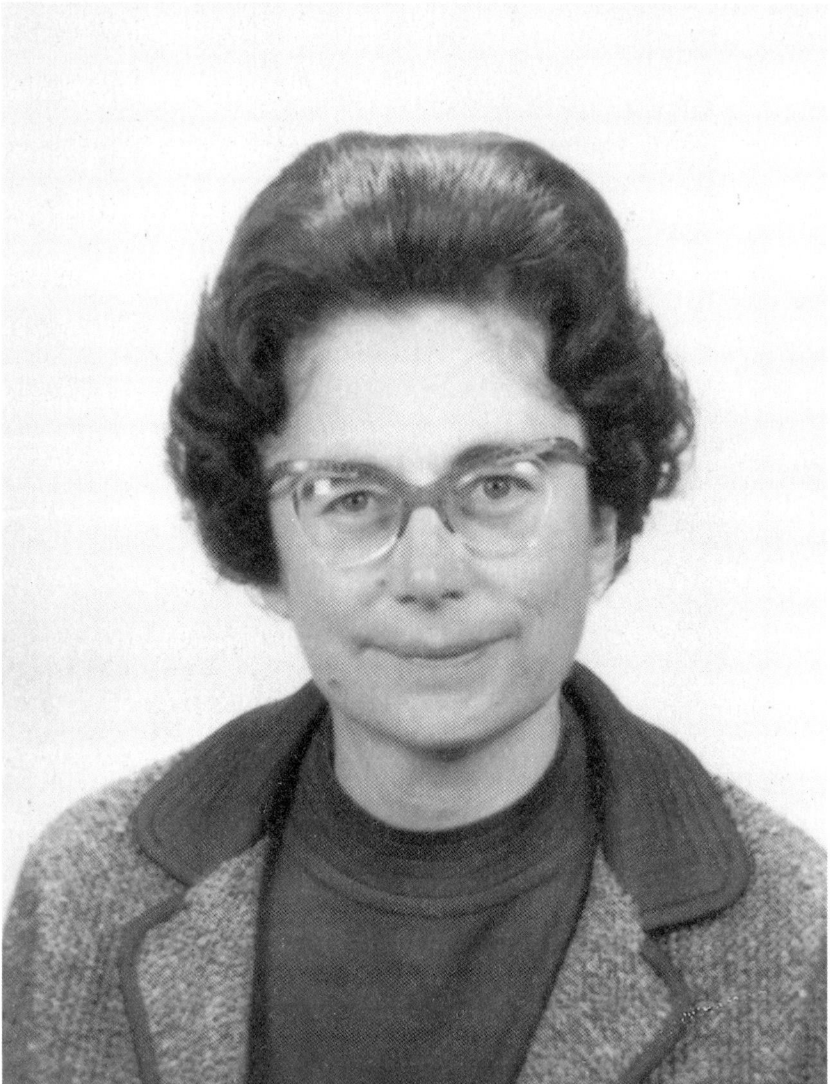

Catrin Williams. FRCS
Hon. Chairman of the Ménière's Society Executive Committee

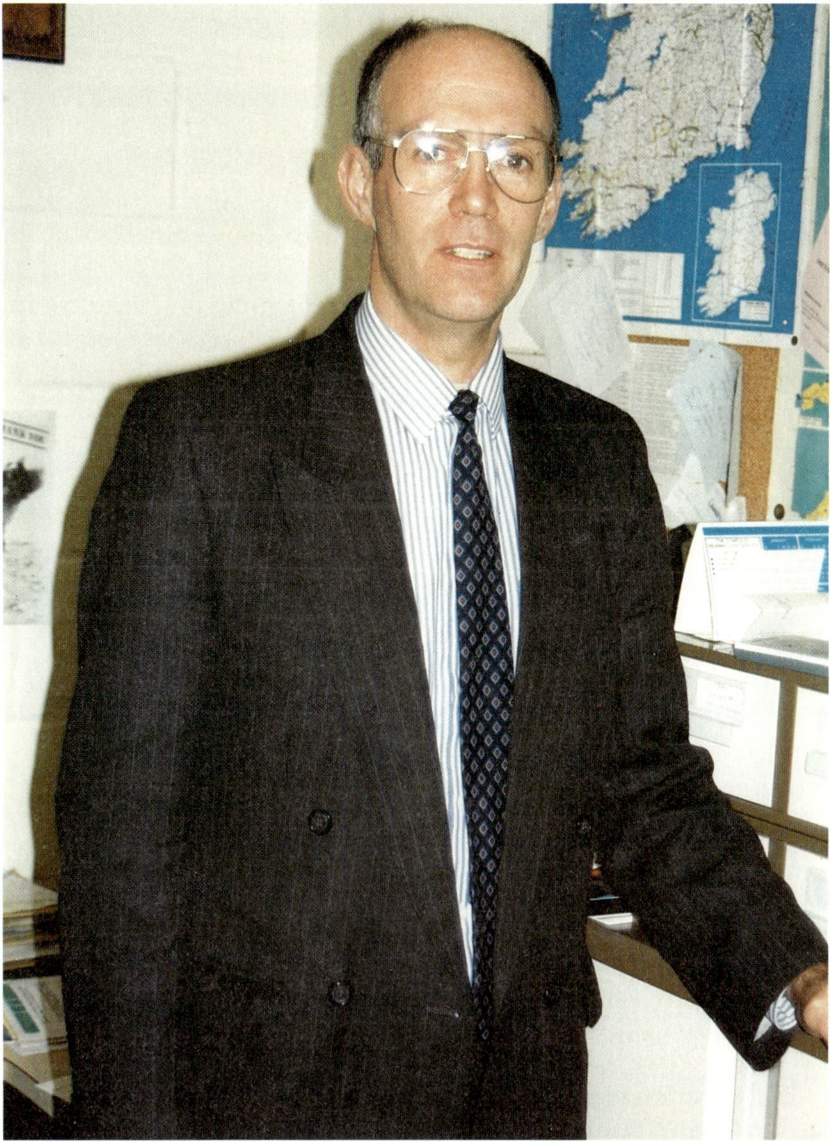

Terry Sheppard
Co-Ordinator of the Ménière's Society

THE MENIERE'S SOCIETY

HELPING YOU "TO LEARN TO LIVE WITH IT"

"You have Ménière's disease and there is no cure. Although there are some things we can do to help, for the most part I'm afraid you will just have to learn to live with it".

Having been told this brutal piece of news by the doctor, just what are the patients' reactions? Probably a state of shock and the inability to digest this frightening piece of news.

For the purpose of encouraging self-help between sufferers and assisting them "to learn to live with it", the Ménière's Society was formed in 1984.

At that time our Founder and Life President was living alone. Her late husband - George La Touche - had been a Ménière's sufferer. She knew what it was like to live with someone having to cope with all the problems the Ménière's syndrome causes but there was no Society then to help her and her husband to 'learn to live with it'.

On one of her international commitments to Holland in 1983 as a voluntary worker for the hard of hearing - she met some Dutch friends who had started a telephone self-help network for Ménière's sufferers. This knowledge created an awareness of what might be possible to explore in the United Kingdom.

With support and encouragement from other hard of hearing colleagues working as volunteers for The British Association of the Hard of Hearing, a limited advertising campaign was undertaken which attracted the attention of the television producers of the programme 'See Hear'. An invitation was accepted to appear on the programme in early 1984 to talk about plans to establish a Ménière's Support Group, from which immediate response came - over 80 letters were received expressing interest within two weeks of the programme. From this beginning of a Support Group, this National and International Society was eventually formed and recognised as a Charity from which time we have never looked back.

Ménière's disease, also frequently known as Ménière's Syndrome, is one of the lesser known conditions and for a person with little or no medical knowledge, easy to understand written information is hard to come by. It is possible that the whole lifestyle of an individual will have to change in order to live something of a normal life and overcome the constant fears.

Sufferers have the fear of recurring attacks when away from home or any assistance; losing a job through continuing absence, - that there will be family upsets, depression, isolation and loneliness; that their credibility may be questioned, - of not being able to keep or make appointments; of letting people down, and of communication problems when there is deafness.

As soon as a diagnosis is confirmed, counselling by a person with experience of Ménière's is of great help to patients and their families. There are patients who become suicidal because they feel alone with this condition and see their life in ruins. Others are angry and frustrated: "Why has this happened to me?" or "It's not fair, I'm still young and starting a good career", or the bitterly disappointed, "I've been so looking forward to my retirement, why am I not going to be allowed to enjoy it?" There is the rejected mum or dad, husband or wife, who because of repeated illness, often at inconvenient times, creates the feeling of "Oh no, not that again!"

It can be equally hard on the family of the sufferer who can only stand by and feel helpless. They will be hit just as hard by the frustrations of cancelled holidays, the ruined Christmas, or "Will he/she be brought home in an ambulance again?"

Many forms of treatment have been effective in lessening the symptoms and bringing about longer periods of relief between attacks, but like all ailments and because no two patients with Ménière's are alike, some drugs suit one person and not another. The emotional make-up of the individual is important and good support from family and friends worth its weight in gold.

Considering all this, the main aims of the Society became assistance, support, cure; the Aims & Objectives becoming:-

The Ménière's Society has been formed for the express purpose of helping those with the symptoms of Ménière's disease which are:- Vertigo, Tinnitus and increasing deafness. We aim to help sufferers to cope with their problems by circulating information and encouraging self-help between members. Additional support may be achieved by means of the following':-

1. To encourage research into manifestations of this disease as it affects different people.

2. To circulate to members from time to time any information on advances that have been made in this field. The issue of newsletters containing the experiences of members and how they cope with their problems.

3. To encourage contact between members by correspondence, telephone or, where possible, by visits.

4. To co-operate with other organisations both here and abroad, having similar objectives.. . .

The Ménière's Society is now a registered charity and is governed by an Executive Committee which is elected by the members. Although the Committee makes the major policy decisions, the day to day running of the Woking based office is in the capable hands of Terry Sheppard, the Co-Ordinator. Being a long term Ménière's sufferer himself he has first hand knowledge and experience of the problems other sufferers so often ask about.

The office operates five days a week, and in addition to Terry, we now have a part time secretarial assistant and two regular volunteers, John Myall and Shirley Harvey, both long term Ménière's sufferers.

When people contact us and say how relieved they are to know we exist, to receive information they can understand, and know they are not alone in the world with their horrible symptoms, it reaffirms that the Society is doing a worthwhile job.

USEFUL ADDRESSES

Association for Teachers of Lip-reading to Adults
The Information Officer
c/o The Post Office
Slimbridge, Gloucester

British Association for the Hard of Hearing
7/11 Armstrong Road
Acton, London
W3 7JL
Tel. 081-743 1110/1353

British Tinnitus Association
Room No. 28
14 - 18 West Bar Green
Sheffield, Sth. Yorks.
S1 2DA

DIAL UK
(National Association of Disablement Information and Advice Lines)
Victoria Buildings
117 High Street, Clay Cross
Chesterfield, Derbyshire
S45 9DZ
Tel. Chesterfield (0246) 250055

National Association of Deafened People
103 Heath Road
Widnes, Cheshire
WA8 6NR

Royal National Institute for the Deaf
105 Gower Street
London
WC1E 6AH
Tel. 071-387 8033

or consult your local telephone directory for:

Social Services
Job Centre
DSS
Local Library

Overseas groups in constant contact with the Society:

Australian Tinnitus Association
c/o Better Hearing
29 West Parade
East Perth, 6004
Western Australia
Contact: Sheila Hittich

Danmark's Meniéreforening
Abildgardsparken 20
3460 Birkerod
Denmark
Contact: Birgit Elk Larsen

Ménière's Australia Inc.
PO Box 202
Moonah
Tasmania, 7009
Australia
Contact: Mrs.V.Barton

Ménière's Support Group of Australia
7 Collinson Road
Cranbourne
Victoria, 3977
Australia
Contact: Mr.A.Tully

SHHH
7800 Wisconsin Avenue
Bethesda
Maryland, 20814
USA
Contact: B.G.Harris

Vereniging Van Ménière-Patienten
Weikantstraat 9
Vilvoorde, 1800
Belgium
Contact: Mr.& Mrs.W. De Hertogh-Jonckeere

Vestibular Disorders Association
1015 N.W. 22nd Avenue
Portland
Oregon, 97210-3079
USA